# THE JOURNEY IS EVERYTHING

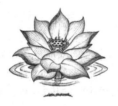

## Saying Yes to Cancer
*Reflections and Inspirations Along the Healing Path*

## SUZETTE HODNETT

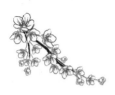

Suzette's book is an inspiring light illuminating the power of love, faith, gratitude, meaning, and stillness in facing cancer, or any challenge. She shares her heartfelt reflections and wisdom, offering us a compass to healing. Moment by moment, breath by breath, she opens her heart and says yes, finding the pearls within the seemingly hardened shells of life.

Gerald Jampolsky, MD and Diane Circicione, PhD
Authors: *Aging is an Attitude*

I have had the privilege of treating cancer patients at a national academic cancer center, and I have witnessed patients and their families navigate through their diagnoses and treatments. Each of these journeys is characterized by the patient's unique personality, life experiences, support system and world view.

From the moment Suzette and I first discussed her diagnosis of cancer, it has been evident to me that she has an immense capacity for love, beauty and tranquility. Her book is an eloquent and fresh perspective of embracing the journey with peace. Her peace does not emanate from accepting her diagnosis with passivity, as she has been intimately involved in understanding, researching and pursuing the best treatment options. Rather it removes the pressure related to the often binary view of cancer treatment, resulting in either remission or relapse. This outlook will undoubtedly help cancer patients find peace in an otherwise tumultuous period, and I am proud to have been involved in her care.

I look forward to reading of the lives helped by this insightful book.

Robert Kang, MD, MPH
Otolaryngology-Head & Neck Surgery, Assistant Clinical Professor
City of Hope National Medical Center, Duarte, CA

The wisdom, love, and insight within Suzette's powerful and positive words offer us the ultimate perspective on how to ride the waves of cancer, or any challenging life circumstance, with meaning, an open heart, and a courageous and calm spirit, connecting us to deep healing and also to each other.

Suzanne Barone, MA, RMT, Director of Complementary Medicine
Presbyterian Intercommunity Hospital, Whittier, CA

First published 2017

ISBN 978 0 692 75445 0

IngramSpark Publishing
New York, New York

Format and Typesetting
Suzette Hodnett
justyourtype.biz

Cover Design:
Suzette Hodnett
Heartstone Arts, Sioux Bailey-Maloof

Cover Photography:
Mike Pellinni

Printed in the United States of America

Library of Congress Control Number: 2017901016

First Edition, January 2017

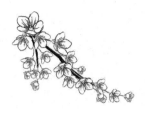

DEDICATED TO

my family
and Team Suzette
who carried me on the wings of their love

and

my sweet feline angel, Tattoo,
who taught me lessons of great calm and courage
in the face of illness

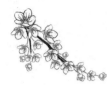

# TABLE OF CONTENTS

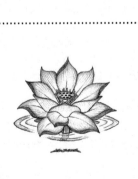

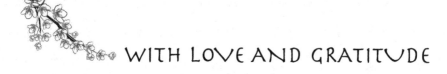

# WITH LOVE AND GRATITUDE

To my family, for taking this journey with me and being such a large part of the miracle of my healing. For their outpouring of great selfless love, immense generosity, and endless compassion. For allowing my life to become their lives and for being my eyes, arms, and engine with an open heart and without a wink of hesitation.

To Team Suzette, for every prayer, positive thought, kindness, generosity, and word of encouragement. For all their deep and continuing love that opened my mind, body and heart to receive all the healing energy.

To my dojo, Aikido-Ai of Whittier, and my sensei, Frank Mc Gouirk, for making me an absent yet ever-present energy surrounded by the warm and tender embrace of their healing chi, generosity, and love.

To sweet Tattoo, for her spirit of unconditional love, peace, joy, and healing, which surrounded me during her life here and beyond the veil.

To my surgeons, Dr. Robert Kang and Dr. Eliie Maghami, for their calm, focus, expertise, artistry, pro-active energy, and the fourteen hours in surgery focused on going for a cure. A special thank you to Dr. Robert Kang for his compassion, present-moment connection, patience, listening spirit, and open heart as we traveled this path together.

To my radiation oncologist, Dr. Sampath, for his continuing tender honesty, great knowledge, kind spirit, and skillful precision. To all the staff in his department, with special gratitude to my radiation therapists, Samantha Garbo and Bridgitt Kibby, for their compassionate touch, open hearts, warm smiles, true concern, and beams of positive thought both in and out of the tunnel. To the receptionist, Barbara Padilla, who welcomed me with such empathy and kindness.

To Dr. Katherine Huang, who reconstructed my eyelid with great skill and kindness, which allowed me the freedom to remove the pirate patch.

To Dr. Auayporn Nademanee, for her care and expertise in guiding my triumphant journey with transformed follicular lymphoma.

To Belinda Torrez, my occupational therapist, whose tender, skillful, and healing touch, compassionate heart, and love kept me buoyed week after week during my treatment.

To my physical therapy team, Ron Vanderbrink and Carla Dunham, who took me through "pain and torture" to greater movement and strength with skill, humor, encouragement, and positive thought.

To City of Hope for saving my life. To every person who works there who met me with an uplifting smile, patient heart, and kind spirit, which made my journey one of light and love.

To President Obama for the Affordable Care Act, allowing me to secure insurance for my preexisting condition and to be seen at City of Hope.

To my dermatologist, Dr. Rachel Moore, for her keen and skillful eye, proactive spirit, and kind heart.

To all of God's creatures, who brought me such joy and peace as I sat in healing stillness in my backyard—the tiny goldfinches, sparrows, and doves, along with all the whimsical squirrels, especially Sweet Pea.

To nature, for its lessons and reminders of rebirth, renewal, and that there is truly a time and purpose to everything under heaven.

To all those that urged me to write this book. Thank you for your inspiration, confidence, and encouragement.

To all of those "beyond the veil"—my best friend Chuck, my parents, grandparents, aunts, uncles, cousin, friends, and the healing angels and guides who continually surround me with their love and peace.

To the infinite loving presence of many names but only one source, for the miracle of my healing and allowing me to be a testimony to the power of love, faith, and gratitude in this world.

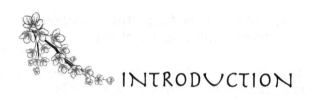

# INTRODUCTION

This is not a book about illness, but about great love, gratitude, and miracles. It is about saying yes and not no, light and not darkness, and great opportunities and not great insults. It is a journey of the heart and not of the body. It is one of opening in trust instead of contracting in fear. It is one of learning and growing, not resisting and resenting. It is my journey, and it is the journey of Team Suzette.

Perhaps the triumph over cancer, or anything, is not measured in the number of our days, but the openness of our hearts during this mysterious, majestic, magnificent, and often messy journey we call life. How much love, light, meaning, and gratitude can we bring to whatever time we are given? No matter what our life challenges are, to truly dance to the rhythm and pulse of God. To somehow, with all our humanity, keep opening time and time again to allow our light to shine. For if our heart closes during any journey, then we have traveled nowhere and learned nothing.

In the blink of an eye, our diagnosis can detour our once seemingly predictable and planned footsteps in the direction of unforeseen vistas and treacherous paths. With a magician's sleight of hand, the cards of our life are now shuffled differently, and we ask in surprise and shock, "What happened?" Our breath, another sunrise, and the number of hellos and goodbyes before our final farewell are no longer taken for granted as our gears now jam in the stark light of diagnosis.

We all walk through our lives in a hypnotic trance until something comes along that grabs us by the shoulders and shakes and wakes us to stare face-to-face with reality. Then the delicate thread of our life is felt deeply, as if for the first time. Not unlike a seamstress carefully reeling the silk, we are reminded of how easily this precious gift can be snapped away from us. We sense the ominous breath of the diagnosis on the nape of our neck, reminding us of our fragility and impermanence, sending chills down our spine.

We enter diagnosis, staging, treatment, or any challenging life circumstance, and tend to put our sights on the future. Our lives will begin once chemotherapy ends, we feel better, and are back to work. We live in waiting for some desired outcome. We want to double and triple jump over our challenges to an imaginary finish line. However, the journey is everything. If we are looking at some optical illusion of a desired end, we don't feel and experience the blessings and lessons that are right before us. We miss the present moment that is our lives: the moment that feels like the neck of the hourglass but that also widens into eternity.

To let the world in takes courage. To experience our physical and emotional pain takes great strength. However, it is often our path to discover our true selves from our experiences. We then bring meaning to what is given and allow it to take us deeper and deeper into awakening. Cancer, or any seeming misfortune, can become our teacher. Focusing on recovery, we toss aside what is frivolous and keep what is essential, allowing the light to shine brighter on what is real and true for us. We often add so much that is unnecessary to our lives, and once we peel the layers off, we come to realize what nourishes and sustains us and what creates a heavier burden. The stillness and silence within our own wilderness of healing brings gifts of clarity and knowing.

How do we say yes to cancer? How do we make space when it feels like there is no space left? How does anyone stay open while going to City of Hope every day, where the energy of cancer can linger like an ominous storm cloud? How do we say yes to the drip of chemotherapy, the insult of surgery, the buckle and bolt of the radiation mask, the tidal waves of nausea, the pain in the dark of the night, and the merry-go-round of side effects? The jigsaw puzzle picture of our lives feels as if it has fallen to the ground and scattered into a million pieces.

If we fully embrace what we are given and let go of what we think we need and want, we open up and, moment to moment, allow life and all its healing energy, lessons, and love to flow through us. We can then trust the bigger picture that all is a great gift. Ultimately, the pearls are revealed within the hardened shell of our challenges. We bow to everything as we do to our teacher, without judgment, knowing all is sacred.

It is hard training to keep saying yes and opening up time and time again. However, the closed fist lets nothing in, while the outstretched arm, hand, and heart allows for healing.

I've given lessons on meditation and led retreats on "Finding Calm Within the Chaos." I've practiced tai chi for twenty years, facilitated support groups, and seen countless clients in therapy. I have taken many twists and turns in life, faced some dark nights of my soul, and experienced and learned many lessons. I've been through physical challenges and experienced the body's incredible capacity to heal, as well as the spirit's amazing resilience and strength.

However, the waves of learning keep crashing on my shore. Life always beckons us to a deeper and deeper knowing and experience. We don't cross finish lines. We just continue to grow. It is an end-less journey. I continue to experience that love given returns to us a hundred-fold and the essence of life as giving and receiving this love. Life continues to reveal the deeper movement from form to spirit, the experience of separation as an illusion, the importance of gratitude, joy, and finding meaning in whatever is happening, the body's immense resiliency, and the truth found in trusting the divine in the 360° view of my life. Again and again, I'm learning, falling, and getting up, holding on, letting in, and letting go, and continue to say "yes" to whatever I'm given. Not an easy task in the face of diagnosis, treatment, recovery, or life itself.

I have notebooks full of tests, summaries, reports, and recommendations with my name on them that rival *War and Peace*. They are in a neat and somewhat tidy box revealing the trajectory of my healing journey. However, boxes can become cramped and distorted, wrapping the experience with a tight ribbon and a bow. Yes, they are the facts, the circumstances. But is that my journey? Perhaps it is the external landscape. Yet we should never be confined by the sharp and predictable corners of the box. We need to keep breathing into what is happening and open ourselves, again and again, to the deeper gifts within our journey. It is then that the edges of the box begin to soften, widen, expand, and fade. Diagnoses and predictions disappear and life becomes the beauty of the day-to-day working on being alive, open, and loving.

We all have our stories, though our leading characters may differ. The setting. The props. The conflicts and the resolutions. Yet there is no difference. Our opening is at birth, followed by a series of acts ending with the final curtain.

We all have our challenges. Our triumphs. Our losses and gains. Our yearnings and fears. Our pain and our awe. We stumble. We fall. We rise again. We fall. We laugh, we love, we resist and yet persist. We live and we die. In our humanity we keep trying to make sense of it all.

So this is not just my journey. It belongs to all of us. It is living on this planet. Being human. Moving through, going beyond, sinking deeper, making sense, rising above, experiencing and absorbing, seeking and finding, losing, and then reclaiming. The specifics of my story may be different from yours. However, the challenges we face and lessons we learn along the way transcend individual details. What we do with the brick and mortar of our own stories ripples out to become our human story. The acceptance and meaning we bring to them becomes our great gifts.

This book is not the story in the manila folders that read "Hodnett, Suzette," but in the empty spaces of its pages. It is the bone and marrow of my journey. As Lao Tzu writes...

> Pots are formed from clay,
> but the empty space within it
> is the essence of the pot.

Out of the mud grows the lotus blossom. What follows are fallen petals along my path. They are the words that I brought back home from my days in the wilderness. This is not a "how-to" book. There are many of those written to guide one in their chosen discipline. It is instead a compass pointing in the direction of all things healing. Reflections, inspirations, and lessons from my journey as I step by step, moment to moment, and breath to breath traveled along my path. They are the words of one soul moving through this crazy and unpredictable yet glorious ride of life. It is my testimony to the gifts of love, gratitude, and miracles received along the way. If it helps one soul navigate their own seemingly treacherous waters to a calmer shore, then I am honored and grateful.

The journey is everything. The glory is in each unfolding day. As the renowned Buddhist monk Thich Nhat Hanh says, it is "moment to moment letting life flow through us." All of it: the pain, sorrow, joy, triumphs, fears, wonder, beauty, and love. We need only to keep saying yes and open our hearts.

Right here, right now.

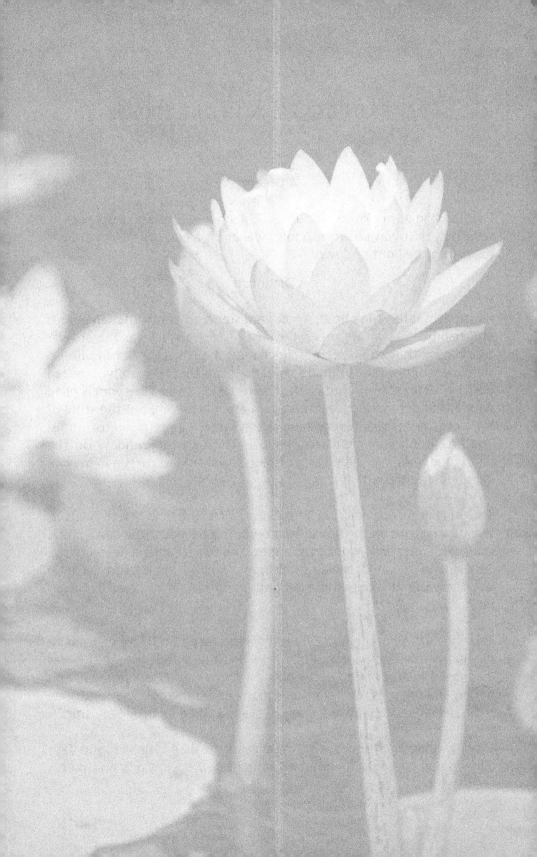

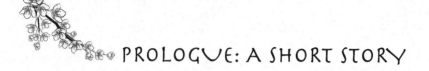

# PROLOGUE: A SHORT STORY

A brief view of the external landscape.

## A Dream

I'm standing at my kitchen counter. The phone rings and a doctor tells me yes, it was positive. A jolt awakens me and the dream disappears into the light of dawn.

## A Diagnosis

Six months later, the phone rings. I am standing at my kitchen counter. I had been awaiting this call every day for a week for the answer to a biopsy that could seemingly change the trajectory of my life. A simple yes or no. The surgeon's voice confirms that the test was indeed positive. After three minutes, the conversation ends. The room is filled with a thunderous silence. I feel as if I am in a dream, but the sting of his words burns real. Everything is the same. The refrigerator hums. The afternoon sunlight casts shadows through the window on the hardwood floor. My kitty Tattoo meows, wanting to curl up in my lap. Yet all feels different.

The tidy jigsaw puzzle of my life is knocked to the floor. Pieces scatter. The new picture on the box is unknown. The kaleidoscope of my mind spins with questions, concerns, hopes, and fears. I take a deep breath. Tattoo licks my hand, the air filter blows, and it is time to go teach tai chi. There remains only this moment. Everything has changed. Or has nothing changed?

Tattoo is sitting on my lap. She is my soft place to fall, my warm cuddle bunny. My companion. Full of unconditional love. When she was diagnosed with severe hypertrophic cardiomyopathy, enlarging lymph nodes, and seizures several years ago, what did she do? She continued to chase bugs, eat, play with her toys, and cuddle up inside my shirt.

How do I become friends with the face of the diagnosis? I spend days allowing all to begin to simmer and digest, weaving bits and pieces from the internet into a space and scenario that offers me peace and comfort.

I remember time and time again. Breathe. All I need is just this moment. All I have is just this moment. I am fine.

I am on a trajectory of appointments, tests, scans, bone marrow biopsies, and second opinions. There's finally a label: Stage Three Follicular Lymphoma, good news and bad news. The good news is that it tends to be a more slowing cancer. The bad news is it is considered incurable, because no treatment has provided a complete remission. The first of many choices: Start immediately with treatment or wait until symptoms develop that beg for relief? Watch and wait it is. I take charge with a regimen to give my body, mind, and spirit all the loving, healing energy to return to perfect health. Goal: Keep all those buggers at bay forever with no need for treatment.

Every three months I am monitored. Life goes on. I teach, train, create art, and see clients. The diagnosis rides shotgun with me.

## The Detour

One year passes with flying colors. I am dancing with the lymphoma in perfect harmony. Then, an enlarged lymph node appears in front of my ear and under my jaw. They are growing, fast. The oncologist feels that the lymphoma has transformed into an aggressive type. There is a party happening inside my head and neck, and they keep inviting all of their friends. More hear about it and come to visit. More tests. A CT/PET scan. Biopsies. A new diagnosis. Advanced metastasized squameous cell stage four cancer. Perhaps inoperable as the scan reveals not only head and neck tumors but activity in the base of the skull.

Each visit the nurse utters disbelief at how fast it's all growing. Sleep is a distant memory as pain becomes a more constant reality. I wonder if the neighbors hear my middle-of-the-night wailing and think I am in pain, or having wild orgasms.

The Tumor Board decides that it is feasible to perform major surgery and go for a cure. Three specialist surgeons are to combine their skill and expertise. They are not sure what they will find or what will need to be done to carve out healthy margins. Definitely a radical neck dissection, but also possible facial paralysis, spinal accessory nerve damage, a missing ear, and assorted invasions into muscles and nerves. Whatever needs to be done will be done.

The unwelcome visitors take up an even larger area of residence. My proactive surgeon sees me two weeks before surgery, and in her concern and knowing, juggles all the logistics and is able to reschedule surgery for a week earlier. Life is both a blur and at a standstill.

Three days before the surgery my sisters create a Team Suzette website to give updates, raise money for medical expenses, and leave guest book messages. The outpouring of love and generosity is humbling and overwhelming. The night before my surgery, I post that "the next chapter of my life is a 'don't know' (as always), but what I do know is that love heals, so I am already healed. Since life is ultimately about how much love we can all give and receive, I feel so very much alive at this precious moment."

Tidal waves of love, positive thoughts, expressions to help, prayers, and good spirits flood through every cell of my body. I go to sleep saying a simple but profound prayer: "Thank you."

## Cut and Paste

The next morning, the surgeons arrive and, after taking one look at me, realize how fast the visitors have continued to grow. My face has already started to become paralyzed from tumor invasion. I see a concerned look in their eyes and ask, "Are you still willing to operate?" One says with a quiet confidence, determination, and kindness: "We are here. We will do everything we can. We will still go for the cure."

I say a prayer: "I am open to the miracle. I am at peace. I am loved. I am healed. I am in God's hands. Thank you."

For fourteen hours, I am under. My family is caught in the limbo of waiting and not knowing. They check the surgery board as if I am a plane running late for arrival. The surgeons and God are my copilots.

I awake with constraints on my arms and legs, breathing tubes, and an inability to talk or move. I keep moving toward the light, if only a memory. The compassionate hand of the intensive care nurse rests on my arm and offers me a sip of water. She covers me with a warm and nurturing blanket of compassion and expertise. We are one as she becomes an extension of all I cannot do for myself.

I am carved and gutted like a Halloween pumpkin. Flaps of fifty lymph nodes have been removed. My jugular vein is cut, my TMJ bone is spliced, my muscles are diced, my face is half-paralyzed, and my spinal accessory nerve is severed. I'm missing an ear like Van Gogh. My right arm is soon to be in a sling, and my eye is covered by a patch. I'm embroidered like my grandmother's favorite quilt, with a large skin graft from my thigh covering the side of my face, neck and lower skull, and I have a partially shaved head. The muscle and nerve pain seems never-ending.

One of my surgeons now stands by my side. I can't talk, but I pull him down to kiss him on the cheek in gratitude and respect. Later, the other surgeon arrives with a report. They are waiting for the pathology findings, but she shares how they were able to get clear margins on the head and neck. The most challenging area was at the base of the skull, as the tumor was already pressing up against it and rapidly advancing upward. They removed as much as possible, but they were impeded by the narrow opening of the jugular vein and could not follow it into the base of my skull. Only so much could be sanded down and still maintain its integrity. My family listens on.

Six Days in a Hospital Gown

My nerves shoot like fireworks in the night sky. Blazes of lightning and currents of electricity jolt through me. I want to move my head side to side but cannot. I rest on my back, turning my head only slightly as hospital staff and family come to visit.

Nurses take me for my first walk. It helps the firing of the nerves to move with the seemingly trapped energy. The next walk I take is with my nephew, who holds my hand and says, "I would take this pain from you if I could."

I make my way to the bathroom and the mirror catches me unaware. The face in the reflection is inflamed, paralyzed, distorted, grafted, and stitched. Perhaps this is a dream. I feel the cold linoleum floor beneath my feet. No, this is the new reality.

I take charge of whatever I can and surrender to what I can't. I refuse shots and pills, but must take others. Sleep is a distant relative. Constant interruptions by the nurses snap me out of any momentary relief I find by relaxing into my breathing. I take joy in the caress of the hospital bed, which bends and lifts in different positions to accommodate me. My family brings in the food they know I would want to nourish and sustain me: organic vegetable soup, organic soft-boiled eggs, and my beloved avocados.

I need fresh air. I plan a great escape. My sisters escort me past the closed doors, down the elevator, through the lobby, and out into the night air. Strong winds wrap around me like the loving arms of a mother. I expand into the endless night sky. The sights and sounds of the outside world collide with the sterile, tiny world of the hospital room. Which is real? I return with leaves on my blanket, dragging it behind me like a wedding dress. I am found out by the nurses. They tell me no fresh air without doctors' orders. I long to be home, and each day I ask: "Today?"

## Home Sweet Home

The days are long. The nights are longer. I revel in stillness and silence. Drains, patches, tubes, sling, stitches, and the continuing fireworks of nerves and muscles are my daily companions. I imagine them all against an expansive star-studded night sky and caressed by a gentle breeze. Noise, jolts, talking, and questions are not my friends. Sleep visits in ten minute intervals, if I'm lucky.

Each time I awaken to the pain, electricity, tightness, throbbing, numbness, and drains, I am reminded, again and again, of what is so right here, right now.

My face feels like it went fifteen rounds with Muhammad Ali in his prime. The now rented hospital bed that supports my body in the best position remains a comfort and salvation.

Moment to moment. Sunrise to the deep dark of the night. My life exists from bed to bathroom, from bed to patio chair. The backyard is my world, my sanctuary, my companion, and my healer.

I spend hours upon hours in meditative stillness. Pillows are propped under my arms to support my head, neck, and shoulders so as not to aggravate either side. The simple turning of my head right to left feels like I am trying to open a jammed door. I sleep in the same pose each night. My right arm remains in a sling and I only use my left side minimally. A half cup of water in a paper cup seems like I am engaged in an Olympic weightlifting event. The patch on my right eye shifts my vision and I walk slowly and precariously. A slight movement can trigger the electric lightning bolts. I feel blessed that I have trained so long in tai chi and can work with the breath. Inhale, exhale. Just right here, just right now.

My house looks like a medical supply store. I look like an infomercial for all its products.

I am a dependent toddler in the arms of my family. I let go of "my way" of doing everything. They are my eyes, arms, and engine. My house is rearranged to be more user-friendly for them and, ultimately, for me. The rotating parade of my dear family empties my drains, cleans and dresses my wounds, shops for and cooks my food, and brightens my yard with fresh flowers, chimes, and bird feeders. Everywhere I look, I see and feel their love and compassion.

Everything feels trapped in a small space in my head and neck, as if pistons keep firing with no place to go. The accelerator is stuck. I walk outside my house at dawn, ever so slowly and precariously, to try to release some of the sensations through movement. I surrender to the expansive light of a new day.

Every day I am read messages from the guest book on the Team Suzette website. I cherish each loving card that arrives to fill my mailbox. My family opens gifts from my them that fling my heart wide open. Prayers, positive thoughts, and encouragement for a full recovery seep into every cell.

I rest in gratitude for small but huge things: any softening of the pain, a pillow placed gingerly behind my back, my vision (although blurred), and removing my medical wristbands. I'm thankful to be eating, if only mush through my mouth's ever-so-small opening. I delight in the flight of the birds and inhaling fresh air instead of the sterile atmosphere of the hospital. I'm missing an ear, but following in the footsteps of one of my favorite artists, Vincent Van Gogh.

Time loses all meaning. Days fade into weeks. One step at a time. Silence comforts me. Birds chirp. A breeze blows. A flower blooms. I believe in the miracle of my healing.

### The Crazy, Lazy, and Hazy Days of Summer

It is only four weeks after the surgery and I receive a call: They are eager for me to start treatment. Usually, the wait is at least eight weeks after such a major surgery before beginning radiation and chemotherapy, so wounds can start to heal and the body can gain some strength. However, they remain proactive due to the aggressiveness of the disease and decide to begin treatment after only four weeks.

My lower eyelid is drooping dangerously from paralysis and scarring. The patch over my right eye must be worn 24/7 to protect the cornea from drying and blindness. The eye does not blink. The hope is to perform a surgery to raise the lower lid to give me the freedom to remove the patch during treatment. Their attempt is unsuccessful. Alas, the pirate look continues as a more invasive operation and skin graft will be needed at least six months after the last radiation treatment.

At four weeks, the show must go on, one step in front of the other. The trifecta of surgery, radiation, and chemotherapy is underway. My body longs for the healing stillness of my home and to gently move through the day at my own pace. However, all now moves relentlessly forward, propelled by the engine of treatment and steered by the doctors. I have a new path: home, to City of Hope, then back again. Day after day.

I meet with the radiation oncologist. He says that they threw the kitchen sink at me in terms of surgery. However, the remaining cancer infiltrated the canals that run along the blood vessels and nerves that go into the brain. They couldn't continue the surgery, or it would have put me at risk. What remains at the base of my skull is more challenging for radiation, but they will focus on that area as well as the entire right side of my face, neck, and skull underlying the graft. I feel deeply at this moment in time that all will be perfectly healed. A full recovery is coming! I have lots more loving, laughing, living, and learning to do! This is just a few chapters in the unfolding, long story of my life.

I'm fitted for a radiation mask that will cover my chest and entire head. It will be bolted down to the conveyor so there is no movement while I'm in the tunnel. Gobs of slippery goo smother and suffocate my face, neck, and chest as they fit me for the mask. I pretend I am at a state-of-the-art sauna in Switzerland, getting a new facial treatment. I return in several days. My alter ego has turned into a neon-green hard plastic mask filled with tiny holes.

Every day I make the journey to City of Hope. I feel as though I am in some kind of bizarre torture chamber as they buckle the mask down tighter and tighter before I enter the radiation chamber. My graft splits open and bleeds, my shoulder screams, my face feels squashed, and it is hard to breathe. I am trapped. No, only if I allow myself to be. The therapists are tender and compassionate. They guide my hair gently outside of the mask, check in with me, and reassure during my time in the tunnel. I just breathe.

I wonder how anyone who has the slightest claustrophobia could ever do this. They tell me: "Heavy drugs, and some refuse." I enter the tunnel with a prayer. I relax every muscle. Focusing on time is my enemy and so it is moment to moment. I imagine myself at my beloved Lake Powell, floating on a raft with the towers of red rock caressing me, while the heat of the radiation is the healing sun. All the beams are only reaching the unwanted cells and melting them into a river of healing.

I meet with the occupational therapist who will help with lymphatic drainage and inflammation. It is a small, loving world, as she is a friend and student from my tai chi classes and my workshops. Her deep compassion, healing touch, and skill help to gently buoy me along twice a week.

The physical therapist's evaluation recommends waiting until after treatment to begin any rehabilitation. The complicated surgery has severed critical nerves, muscles, blood vessels, and panels of lymph nodes, and radiation will cause further assault to all the tissue. My arm must remain in the sling. He is thrilled to hear I have such extensive training in tai chi, which will complement his therapy.

I meet with the medical oncologist, who explains this chemotherapy as the most "emetogenic" of the therapies. I hope it means "effective." I look the word up on the Internet and the definition is "most likely to induce vomiting." The handout I am given has a long list of side effects from this chemotherapy. I take a quick glance, fold it in half, and put it away. I will allow whatever unfolds to be my experience.

A few days later, the strange world of chemotherapy begins. The bags are locked in a refrigerator with dual signatures needed for release. I'm given a private room because the infusion is so long. I welcome it as my quiet healing chamber, and the chemotherapy as an elixir to target the unwelcome visitors. I embrace the warm, heated blanket, their special foot slippers, and my subliminal tapes. I picture every drop deeply penetrating and healing every cell. I invite it in to clear everything out to the far side of the moon. I drink water, ask that the lights are off, and rest in healing stillness. Time disappears. They pull out the IV six hours later and tell me it's time to go home.

My sister and sister-in-law pick me up and we "optimize the chemotherapy." A half an hour of exercise is first. I walk with my sister and hold her belt loop for strength, stability, and vision. Five minutes of one foot in front of the other, and then I must rest. A few more minutes and a wave of nausea. Rest. I have to keep moving. At last, the thirty minutes are up. Then, there is a half an hour in a hot bath. At first it is welcoming, but soon the heat feels suffocating. I picture the cells opening to receive the river of chemotherapy. Eight cups of water are placed on the rim of the bathtub like toy soldiers. I do my best to drink them all. Opening. Flushing. Healing. Finally back to bed. My body is pulsating and the waves of nausea rise. I try to ride them as I did the surf in past summers. Wipeout. Days fade into the next, and my life is whatever is right in front of me at the moment. The same, or different?

Telling signs of radiation begin to broadcast themselves in my body. My already compromised jaw closes tighter, so I need a children's Minnie Mouse toothbrush inserted sideways just to reach a few teeth. The skin on my head and neck feel like they may burst like an overinflated balloon, and gradually they begin to look like the bark of an old, charred tree. My mouth is as dry as a desert wind. My taste is metallic and foreign. My throat is sore when I swallow. A new tiredness called fatigue visits.

I continue to wake up throughout the night to the ever-changing sensations in my body and the reality of my life, right here, right now.

I can no longer fit a spoon into my mouth. I now use the "vacuum and suck it up" approach to bring small bits of food into my mouth. The tiny finches slowly eat at their bird feeder with me. They are my companions. We are one, a single tiny peck at a time.

My young nieces and nephews come to visit. They hear my paralyzed speech and look at my distorted face, patch, sling, missing ear, and weakened body, and surround me with their sweet spirits. We sit outside, and since my right arm is immobilized, we all try to write with our left hands. We design art. We laugh. I assure them I'm healing and all will be better. I wonder if they think my ear will grow back.

I am able to maneuver myself independently at night and in the mornings. While my right arm still remains in a sling, I can now use my left hand for extremely light lifting. Baby steps.

Waves of nausea seem to rarely ebb. The slightest movement or talking threatens a crash. Soon I cannot stand to look at my once cherished avocados. I sit in stillness before and after I eat. Mindfully, I create a new and ever-so-slow dance with my food. What works one day drops off the radar the next. My organic veggie pureed soup remains a friend. Sometimes my body tells me it is best to not eat at all.

My life is a tunnel. I reach out for the light and trust that it is just beyond the darkness. I find joy in the morning symphony of the birds, the tender hand of the radiation therapist on my back, gently holding the belt loop of a loved one, the changing shadows on my lawn, Hotei's ever-smiling face in my backyard, and the return home each day to cards and doorstep deliveries.

I believe in the miracle of my healing.

# Halfway: The Unwelcome Node Biopsy

I reach the halfway mark. I feel a swollen node under my chin. Is it scar tissue? The lymphoma? A few squameous cells that have jumped the fence and ended up on the other side of the carved canyon? The unwelcome node biopsy is done. It is confirmed: Yes, a straggler. It is critical that the area at the base of my skull not have a break in treatment with surgery. They will expand the area of radiation and lengthen the treatment time and duration. By the next day, my proactive radiation oncologist has adjusted and widened the area. The show must go on.

Time has lost all meaning. I am no longer crossing days off a calendar. I don't notice it anymore, as I often make my way straight to a horizontal position on my bed, or sit in stillness in the patio chair.

Talking and movement rock the boat. It is as if I have a perennial case of the worst flu or food poisoning. My beloved dojo is having a Team Suzette fundraiser/seminar in the park. My spirit so longs to be there, but my body speaks loudly to remain in the horizontal position.

My right arm remains in a sling, and the patch is still on my right eye. My perspective is off, so I bump into walls and walk into the sliding screen door. I write a little, albeit carefully and slowly, with my left hand. Minimal movement allows for less upset of the graft, less pain, and better healing of my muscles and nerves.

Each day I rise and know that the show must go on. I put one foot in front of the other.

I keep finding joy and gratitude amid this new world. I open my heart to receive everyone's gracious gifts of time, energy, and love. My family is my safety net in the world. I am a toddler leaning on them for support. I revel in what I can do and let go of what I can't.

I feel like I should wear a sign around my neck that says: "Beware! Toxic Waste Dump!"

Sleep plays a massive game of hide and seek—mostly hide. I long to stretch out under the covers in all directions, but it is not possible with the challenges from the severed spinal accessory nerve and sling. I find the best pose and don't move throughout the night.

One step at a time. Connecting with my breath sometimes keeps the tide from rising higher and the wave of nausea from crashing. The energy work I know how to do on myself focuses, balances, and opens me.

Eating becomes increasingly more difficult, and it's not just from the nausea. The already tiny opening of my mouth from paralysis and severing of the TMJ joint is being compromised further from the fibrosis of the radiation. The food goes in the hatch. The food falls out of the hatch. I'm definitely not ready for luncheon guests.

It is a bumpy road, but I keep all my arms and legs inside the vehicle, and my seat belt is my breathing, everyone's love, and giving my body the time and space for this current road trip.

At night I am alone. I enjoy the quiet, but sometimes in the deep, dark of the night, I so long for a hand to hold, another heartbeat next to mine, or a soft healing touch.

My best friend one day in the food department is my worst enemy the next. I listen to my body and have it tell me what I can and can't handle moment to moment.

In the final weeks of treatment, I am constantly riding the waves of nausea. I have lost all contact with my stomach. Stillness is the blanket I wrap around me to help lower the tide. All other side effects ride piggyback on the nausea. I move slowly and mindfully. Everything is a reminder to take nothing for granted and to find joy in what would seem like even the smallest of gifts.

Time becomes meaningless in the face of illness, surgery, treatments, and recovery. In my art studio, ten hours could seem like ten minutes. For the last three months, time has stood still. Just moment to moment, breath to breath, and step to step.

I take nothing for granted and surrender to everything. The highlight and joy each day is arriving home to loving cards and doorstep deliveries from Team Suzette that fling my heart wide open. My family reads them to me. I hold them tenderly in my left hand and gaze through one blurred eye. I dictate updates, thoughts, and gratitude to my sisters, who post my words on the Team Suzette website.

Each day I return to the radiation tunnel, each week to the drip, drip, drip. Moment to moment. One day I am given a medal that says "champion." I feel like I deserve it. The "next appointment" slip they hand to me has a four letter word: "None."

My sisters and nephews take me on a celebratory stroll to the end of the Seal Beach pier to watch the sun set in the sky and on my treatment. A few weeks later, a CT scan of my head and neck is taken to observe the state of the new nodes that came to visit halfway through my treatment. All else cannot be accurately determined until several months after treatment. Hallelujah! The scan reveals that the new nodes did a disappearing act. However, it also shows "suspicious nodes" remaining under the graft, although smaller.

Another decision rests in my skinny little lap, two options. Due to the past aggressiveness of the unwelcome visitors, the Tumor Board suggests aggressive surgery to remove the lymph node panel containing the suspicious nodes under the grafted area. This option contains the risk of infection, cutting through blood vessels that support the healing graft on my face, and more trauma to my body. The second option is to wait one month for the scheduled CT/PET scan to see if these particular nodes have continued to shrink. The risk is that they would throw another wild party in the meantime and invite all their friends.

I decide against the knife. A vote of confidence goes to my body to continue to kick everything to the far side of the moon through prayer, positive thought, everyone's love, Divine light, and the results of all the treatments. POOF! All will be gone.

I remain humbled and in deep gratitude to Team Suzette. Everywhere I look I see love in the cards on my table, Mt. Baldy rocks, posters, prayer flags, my bank account, gifts, and uplifting letters and cards of compassion and encouragement. I may be on a very crazy journey, but I also feel like the most blessed person in the world.

I believe in the miracle of my healing.

# FALL

I am a free woman. No longer do I have to make the daily push to City of Hope to be poked, poisoned, and prodded. My body rejoices in unwinding into each day and moving with its own rhythm. The real healing can begin.

I watch an ever-changing parade of symptoms pass through my body each day. This is not a linear journey. My appetite slowly and unpredictably begins to return, but my stomach still feels lost in space. I gain several pounds. Side effects come and go. The only certainty is that everything changes. Sludgy thoughts vacillate between moments of clarity. Ever-changing sensations shift in my head, neck, and shoulder. Moments of small bursts of energy are laced with periods of fatigue. I continue to look at the world with a patch on one eye. My jaw remains partially locked. My right arm is still in a sling. My eye tears, burns, and blurs. I have become a lefty, and maneuver the world with this willing but weaker side. Delicate threads of my own grounded energy play hide and seek. I rest. I unwind. I embrace stillness.

When I arrived home from surgery in May, sunflower seeds were planted in my backyard. They are now blooming! Suzette and sunflowers are rising toward the sun!

It is time for the CT scan to see the state of the suspicious nodes. I decided to allow them to heal on their own versus the aggressive surgery. The scan reveals that they have done a disappearing act. My head and neck surgeon uses words like "encouraging" and "amazing."

I feel as if I am waking up from a dream. I begin to widen my aperture and remember a life before surgery and treatment.

I take longer and longer early morning walks in the light of dawn, often bolting out of bed to move with the seemingly trapped sensations of twisting, burning, and throbbing in my neck and shoulder. I continue to awaken in the wee hours of the night and stand beneath the indigo sky, allowing its expanse to comfort and embrace my body.

Long days of stillness and healing unfold before me in a gentle reprieve. Tiny miracles take center stage.

Little by little, I begin to clean different places in the house and feel subtle shifts in energy. Assorted gauzes, ointments, prescriptions, and and pills I never used are tossed with glee. My house slowly begins to feel like my home again.

A month later, what stares up at me from my plate is more of a welcomed friend. My menu broadens. I have lost sixteen pounds since the onset of chemotherapy (and I was an extremely lean machine before). Avocados now smile up at me from my plate with each meal. The left-handed chef mindfully and slowly cooks three organic, nourishing meals a day. It feels like a full-time job. I still need help cleaning up the dishes, especially the pots and pans. I eat, but remain a work in progress. My taste buds continue to play tricks on me. My mouth does not pry open very wide, so I only get a little down the hatch at a time.

It is time to return to City of Hope for physical therapy. I long for more days of healing at home, not pushing my body once again. Alas, the show must go on.

The sling that has been taking the weight off of my shoulder and neck for the last five months is finally removed. Ah, sweet release. PT (Pain and Torture) begins, and they start by digging deep to loosen my frozen shoulder. I wail like a child as they try to melt the deep freeze. I'm given a Therabite device to try and loosen up the jaw and scar tissue.

I experiment with creating art. Returning to my life as an artist is a big unknown. I hold the scissors gingerly in one hand. I cut and listen to the ensuing conversation in my shoulder and neck. I attempt to reach my arm out far enough to do a little fusing. Baby steps.

The bark-like skin on my neck from radiation begins to soften. The internal scar tissue feels as if it wants to hold its ground. People want to know how, when, and what. I have no crystal ball, and just flow within moment-to-moment realities.

It is time for the all important MRI focusing on the base of the skull. They are unable to confirm any suspicious areas of disease. The radiation oncologist explains that the enhancement patterns/abnormal signals can likely be the result of postoperative and post–radio-therapy inflammatory changes. I embrace his words as great news that the unwelcome visitors remain on the far side of the moon and miracles continue! POOF! I rest in gratitude.

It is one month into the prescribed treatment of physical therapy. Amazing what some pain and torture can do for you. The physical therapist says I am exceeding all expectations. Such small movements seem like such huge miracles. Therapy sessions, tai chi, and disciplined work at home continue to be a winning combination.

My hair starts to return from surgery and radiation. My skin begins to smooth and soften. My ear is still missing, but I'm doing a great comb-over. It is a little easier to maneuver words out of the paralysis. My mouth slowly begins to open a little wider.

Milestones appear.

I return to my dojo to stand before my sensei and all the students and finally thank them in person for their endless love, generosity, kindness, and support over all these months. I am overwhelmed and humbled. I speak from my heart. I lead the class. I love everyone.

A local art exhibition in October, the Harmony Fine Art and Craft Show, lovingly gives me a free booth and offers to set up and staff my exhibit. I attend for a few hours. Many friends come to visit for the first time since my surgery. It feels miraculous to be standing in the midst of my art and among my friends. It is challenging to be there, but worth every nanosecond.

A compassionate neighbor organizes and gives a lecture at a local art gallery with donations going to Team Suzette. I attend and am touched by her gift and a full house of deep love and support.

I join my sister in the Walk for a Cure to support her and her challenges with epilepsy. It is more of a stroll and rest and stroll some more, but it feels magnificent to be supporting her and to be out in a sea of humanity.

I celebrate my birthday with my first overnight voyage out of the house, to Cambria with my sister and her wife. I am so thankful and I absorb the stillness, fresh air, timeless beauty, and peace like a dry sponge.

My sensei asks me to perform a demonstration and share an essay on tai chi to advance in rank to my fourth-degree black sash. I give a talk about tai chi, healing, and love. I do an original exhibition of moves (as best I can with a patch, sling, and limited movement) and feel like a walking miracle. My gratitude and my love permeate each word and fill each move.

The hospital bed disappears. I reclaim more and more of my house. My family of backyard companions continues to grow. Sweet Pea the squirrel arrives and stands on my foot in trust and pleads for a snack. Birds flutter everywhere and we connect in silence.

I am eating more food through my mouth's opening. I'm still not ready for Amy Vanderbilt's etiquette table, but I'm doing better. I'm able to use a fork or chopsticks to guide small quantities into my mouth with a sucking motion.

I'm a work in progress, but making amazing progress. Stamina, fatigue, pain levels, clarity, and sleep are ever-changing. I find joy in the days I can be at my house moving and resting at my own pace. I listen to and nurture my body, letting it reveal the future. What is here today may or may not be here tomorrow.

I continue to revel in all I can do. I teach my Saturday morning tai chi class at the dojo. I spend more and more time creating my artwork. Yes, with adaptations, but isn't all of life a series of adaptations?

It is December and time for a PET scan to look at the whole enchilada. Miracles continue. "No change and no issues." The stinkers are staying on the far side of the moon, where they belong forever! The doctor's words are "Great News! Very encouraging." So far, so amazing. A merry Christmas gift indeed.

I believe in the miracle of my healing.

WINTER

Leaves fall to the ground. I gain more ground. Twelve pounds return to my body. I'm probably the only one who can tell.

How I feel remains as ever-changing as the seasons. My body continues its valiant efforts to heal, balance, ground, and cleanse from being carved, dripped, injected, and nuked. My morning healing regimen grows to include meditation, a morning walk of gratitude, prayer, and reflection, as well as jaw and physical therapy exercises, adapted qigong and tai chi for my body, mind, and spirit, and a nourishing, healthy, organic breakfast.

The body's capacity to heal is phenomenal. I continue to learn how to dance with this new body and its changing sensations. A glance in the mirror or at a recent photo of my distorted, drooping, and embroidered face can still cause the film in my mind to flicker and sometimes jam, burn, and then readjust. The garment of my body has taken on a different form. However, the spirit that I am remains the same and wraps its loving arms around me and the world.

Physical therapy continues. They decide to keep the shoulder partially frozen to help stabilize the area. They work the scar tissue beneath the graft and under my eye to help soften the area to stimulate blood vessels for my possible eye surgery and graft in February.

The wait is over. The oculoplastic surgeon gives me the clearance to have the reconstructive surgery on my lower lid to protect the cornea and remove the patch. She takes skin from my upper arm to move to the eye. She isn't sure of the outcome, but will give it her best. Physical therapy comes to a standstill while I recover from the eye surgery and graft. Humpty Dumpty Hodnett is partially getting put back together again.

My morning walks get longer. I'm teaching more regularly at the dojo and creating art in my studio. I long for days and time uninterrupted to follow my energy without going into too much overdrive and to so many appointments.

Another local art show, the Hillcrest Festival of the Fine Arts, invites me to participate with the gift of a huge, complimentary exhibit space. It is only several days after my eye surgery and graft and I am still recovering, but am very honored and grateful to be there. I wear sunglasses, but underneath, for the first time in almost a year, there is no patch.

With my sling finally removed, I experiment with using my shoulder and neck to cut and fuse my art. I begin with one small, solitary panel that represents a theme along my healing path. Months later, with baby steps, patience, and adaptations, one panel turns into *The Journey is Everything*, a 5.5' × 4.5' artwork consisting of twenty-seven panels forming a 3D mixed-media tapestry reflecting the gifts and lessons along my journey.

I am asked to exhibit my artwork at City Hall for a month. It is uplifting to remain connected to the community as an artist.

In April, I return to teach tai chi at a local community center. Driving is a work in progress, but the Team Suzette beloved friends volunteer to shuttle me for the forty-five minutes to and from the class. I am wiped out the next day, but it feels amazing to stand before a group of new students again. Yes, with a different body, but with an even deeper understanding of tai chi principles from my journey.

The follow-up with the eye surgeon says the skin graft is healing well. She says there is no need for the threatened shots to soften the hardening scar tissue that could pull the graft down.

During my sisters' spring break from school, they graciously invite me to return with them to the healing stillness, magic, and beauty of Cambria. The time and space away from everything, the clean air, and the all-embracing quiet is deeply healing and reminds me of all that is timeless and true. The garment of my body may have changed, but that infinite space connected to everything and everyone remains the same.

I believe in the miracle of my healing.

SPRING

My backyard sanctuary gets a much needed and long drink of water to quench its thirst. Warm blasts of sunny, warm temps follow, and the blossoms, sensing it is their time to join the world again, burst into bloom. So do I.

Everything still changes. How I feel is dependent on how much I sleep, how much my head, neck, and shoulder are talking to me, what I'm doing, what I've done, how much I've had to push and my time to recover, and how often I can move at my own healing pace. I go with the flow of ever-changing currents each day.

It is time for the next MRI to the head, neck, and base of the skull. Pain, challenges in eating and chewing, trismus, physical therapy, and side effects are discussed with the radiation oncologist. Then there's great news: No sign of any unwelcome guests on the head/neck/base of the skull. His word: "Awesome!" What an amazing gift in my Easter basket!

Happy Anniversary! It is May 7 and 12 months have passed since I was under fourteen hours of surgery. It has been a year of challenges and triumphs, of mysteries and miracles. It has been a time of saying yes and moving toward the light and of great insults transformed into great lessons. I may not be what was, but am amazed at what is.

Memorial Day weekend and my dojo's 34th annual retreat to the Mt. Baldy Zen Center is here once again. Last year the retreat seemed as far away as my missing ear. Embraced by the mountain peaks that play hide and seek in the soft, heavenly fog, I return to Mt. Baldy and am surrounded by loving friends, gentle training, and an opportunity to thank everyone for all the love given to me.

My baby steps have somehow slowly become great leaps. I look back at the year and see a beautiful tapestry woven together with gifts of faith, blessings, healing, joy, kindness, generosity, and immense love. It has been challenging in many ways, but inspiring in so many others. The journey has been a testimony to my great doctors, an organic and healthy diet, tai chi, qigong, longer walks, all the love, prayers, generosity, and positive thoughts of the family and friends in Team Suzette, the body's amazing capacity to heal, the spirit's incredible power to rise above, and Divine grace.

I am invited to participate in the two month Laguna Beach Art-A-Fair over the summer. It is a huge undertaking, even without my current realities, but I embrace the preparation one tiny step at a time, along with the help of Team Suzette. I give birth to new, larger artworks inspired by my journey, entitled *One With Everything, Phoenix Rises from the Ashes*, and *Joy*.

I am thankful for the miracle of my healing.

## SUMMER

Amazing grace and miracles continue to unfold with each new chapter of my healing journey.

My morning regime of meditation, walking, tai chi, qigong, and a nourishing breakfast continues and deepens. My backyard sanctuary does cartwheels under the warmth of the sun.

I begin baby steps in writing this book. Team Suzette and I set up my art show at the Laguna Art-A-Fair. I walk along the beach with friends. I create more artwork and seek as many hours as I can in the studio amid doctor appointments, physical therapy, small surgeries, other projects, and teaching several tai chi classes. My clinical follow-up with the head and neck surgeon results in two thumbs up. I am happy. So is he.

At the six-month follow-up with my eye surgeon, she declares the surgery a success and that the healing has been excellent.

I take some beginning drives close to home. My patch is off, allowing for full vision. However, one eye often burns, tears, and blurs from paralysis and a lack of blinking. Challenges remain in my ability to turn my head left or right due to the graft and severing of the nerves. Bone rests on bone, and changing gears without aggravating the nerves and muscles in my neck and shoulder is difficult. Like all else, baby steps are welcomed with gratitude. I'm on the road again.

I am fitted for a custom shoulder brace to hopefully lessen the discomfort in my back, shoulder, and neck. It looks great on the hanger, but they forgot that because of the cutting of the spinal accessory nerve, I don't have enough range of motion and strength to put it on! Back to the drawing board, with the hope that someone is able to think outside of the box to create a special Suzette design.

The opening night of my two-month art exhibit in Laguna Beach is filled with such love, support, and sales!

Several unwelcome critters are found along my skin's surface. Surgeries are underway to excavate them. I am monitored closely to assure that they only dance on the top floor and don't venture underground. Eight surgeries are performed in a marathon of eight weeks.

Doctors continue to talk about what may be the new normal. I continue to just look at each day as what is so in each moment. I create new steps and routines to best dance with the ever-changing energy levels and sensations. I may not be what was, but I am so very blessed by what is. I remain forever grateful for my amazing progress and the miracle of my healing.

Life can seem to speed by in a blur before our very eyes. We can also look back and trace our moment-to-moment experiences. Wasn't it just yesterday I was on vacation in Pismo Beach with my nieces and nephews playing in the surf, burying them in the sand, and taking long early morning walks along the shore? Two months later, I was deep down into a fourteen-hour surgery. Everything changes and nothing changes. It is July a year later. My nieces and nephews come to visit. We go to the beach. I slather on more sunscreen than I ever have in my life. My SPF 50 hat and light clothing cover are my new bikini. I bury their feet in the sand with one hand. I look out to the oncoming waves with one eye burning and tearing. We laugh as the waves crash on us. Same or different? Isn't life grand?

From the ashes rises the phoenix.

This is a very short story. The broad brush strokes of my external landscape for those that want to hear the back story. It is the outward movement in time. As the great spiritual teacher Ram Dass would say, "grist for the mill." The mere circumstances. It is not the story of our life but the meaning we bring to it that reflects our true healing. What follows are the delicate, golden threads that wove the blessed tapestry of my life together throughout this journey: Inspirations, reflections, themes, and remembrances of the love, gratitude, lessons, and miracles that have been my precious gifts along my healing path.

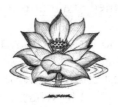

# REFLECTIONS AND INSPIRATIONS
## ALONG THE HEALING PATH

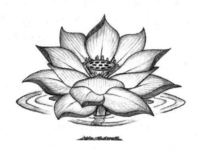

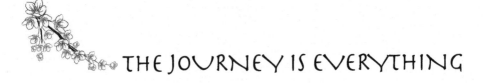

# THE JOURNEY IS EVERYTHING

How much of human life is lost in waiting?
Ralph Waldo Emerson

We must let go of the life we have planned,
so as to accept the one that is waiting for us.
Joseph Campbell

The diagnosis is given and then all sights are set on "getting through" to the end of treatment. We wonder: "When will chemotherapy end?" "When will I return to work?" "When will I feel better?" "When is the point where I can live again?"

It would be so easy to assume a waiting position throughout this healing path, to let it become the theme song of our lives. Waiting for diagnosis, waiting for the next appointment, waiting for the pain to lessen, waiting for energy to return, waiting for test results, waiting for radiation to be over, waiting for the last drip of the chemo bag, waiting to "return" to life, waiting for a five year "cure," waiting for the end of symptoms, and waiting for the "new normal" to return to the "old normal." It is not much different than life itself. We wait for our kids to grow up, for the weekend, for our vacation, for winter to end, for the love of our lives to appear, for the supermarket line to dwindle, for our income to improve, and for retirement to follow our dreams. We keep waiting for our lives to get better until we finally wait for our own death. Waiting can be a dangerous stance, as it puts our lives on pause. Waiting is a rebuke to this moment in time. Whether we wait patiently or impatiently, waiting is a weak position that transforms our lives into a preferred future space and time. No matter where we are, it is always so easy to want to fast-forward to a place of more seeming ease, or rewind the film backward to a place of comfort from the past. Both of these catch us in the limbo of powerless waiting, and deny us the immensity and gift of the present moment.

This is true for all of us no matter what falls upon our path. There is a bump in the road, a needed "detour." We lose whatever prescribed path we thought we were on. Those of us on a healing journey discover that our recovery, just as our lives, is not linear. It bends and flows; the less we flow with it, the more we are seeped in suffering.

Nothing is ever fixed; we are always in a constant state of transition, moment to moment. There is no guarantee nor set of instructions on the box of our life. However, we are great illusionists and trick ourselves into believing that our lives are anchored and unchanging. We long for security and the familiar. It's no wonder that when illness, loss, misfortune, and death come, it is so difficult for us. We do not like the unknown when we are in unchartered land and there is no map. With diagnosis, any seeming comfort and familiarity is gone, and we are catapulted onto a confusing and unknown path. We want to move through the journey from illness to health by crossing over the bridge to the other side, where there are no seemingly treacherous waters below. We want to look at the horizon and not at what is in front of us. We long to be on seemingly safe and solid ground so life can begin again.

Our life is parceled into intervals for the follow-up tests and we are often given predictions of reoccurrence and a prognosis for survival. This MRI is clear, but they need to do another in three months. We may think, what if I only have six months, a year, or five years to live? It is challenging to not want to fast-forward to when chemotherapy is over, radiation is done, tests are taken, our energy returns, and side effects soften into a deeper healed body. However, each step of our journey is sacred and meaningful. Our diagnosis, treatment, and recovery may offer a different view and ground, but nonetheless remain a place to discover great lessons in balance, beauty, and inner strength. It is our precious life right now. We find ourselves asking, "When will this be over?" But often we do not ask the question that is even more huge and foreboding: "What if I'm not here right now?"

Our time of diagnosis and treatment is our time to trust and open up to the unfolding journey, to listen, say yes, commit, be present, and flow with grace into the unknown current of our lives.

It is not always easy. Our recovery is fertile breeding ground for "what ifs." It is challenging not to feel the "weight" of the "wait" after a PET scan, where the results won't be known for a few days and we want and need to know now! We wait in the lobby for the doctor, who is behind schedule again. An hour has already gone by. We keep waiting for our symptoms to disappear and for our pain to lessen. We wait as we cross off all the days on the calendar of treatment. We wait to return to work. Waiting. Waiting. Waiting.

However, the journey remains everything. The journey is moment-to-moment living. The ride has to be as important as the destination, because the ride is our lives, regardless of the peaks or valleys. Bumps in the road, small or seemingly insurmountable, are the stuff that growth is made of. Every moment is a gift and an opportunity to give meaning to our lives.

Each second is an intricate thread in the journey; each drip of chemotherapy, each blast of radiation, each prick of the IV needle, each encounter with our doctors, and each moment of our recovery weaves our healing path together. Our challenges are our times of greatest transformation. The Chinese hànzì for crisis has two symbols: one for danger and one for opportunity. It is so easy to get focused on our new melodrama of pain, fear, and symptoms that we often miss the beauty and gifts interwoven within the tapestry of our journey. And so we miss our life. Mark Twain echoes this brilliantly with his famous quote, "My life is a series of 'what ifs' that never happened."

Who wants to live in the present of the radiation tube, the chemotherapy drip, the nausea, the fatigue, the hope, and the despair? It requires finding meaning and gratitude in what unfolds in front of us. If we continually want to fast-forward to a "better time" and are not present in our lives, then we can't experience the lessons and grow in divine light. Every time we accept, we open a little wider and a little deeper and let in more love, light, and healing. Ultimately, we embrace both the prick of the thorn along with the beauty and the glory of the rose. We rest in stillness. Pay attention. Give thanks. We stop looking forward and then see the miracle of life before us.

I do not want to miss the countless moments of abundant life right here, right now, by defaulting into a waiting game. I cherish the moments of grace given as I sit in healing stillness watching the golden rays from the sun painted against a delicious, deep, blue, and icy canvas of a sky. I embrace the early morning quiet only broken by a symphony of birds. I appreciate the gift of a single robin dressed in a blazing red vest perched on the edge of my patio chair. I am thankful for the dawning of another precious day, a summer morning in pajamas with the sun on my back, and the smell of the newly mowed grass from my neighbor's yard wafting through the window. All the healing love, positive thoughts, gifts, and prayers offered by Team Suzette deepen my healing.

We do not have to like the nausea, the pain, and the dark night of our body. However, we can accept and honor it as what is happening right here, right now. This releases its hold on us. The daily motto of a woman who was going through a heavy schedule of dialysis was, "I am going in for these treatments, but I am continuing with my same happy life."

We are always weaving the tapestry of our lives. We are creating its design one thread at a time. Each thread is important to the whole. Everything matters. If we stay present in the journey, it uplifts and lightens our heart and transforms us. Our healing path is a reminder to stay awake and that each moment is an entryway to the pulse of the infinite.

So what do I do if I'm not waiting? For me, I breathe into the amazing present moment. I feel the miracle of life. I sense my feet on the ground. I soak in the sounds and sensations of what surrounds me. I connect with the person next to me. I give thanks, reflect, center, toss up a prayer, send some love out to someone, and then to everyone. I rest with whatever is, even if it is the now of the bolted radiation mask, the rising wave of nausea, the heaviness of fatigue, and all the "don't knows." The journey asks that we find meaning and gratitude in the path in front of us.

The motion picture screen in my mind rewinds to age seventeen, traveling up the coast to San Francisco in my VW van with two friends. In a bookstore, I found one of the most inspirational and pivotal books: *Man's Search for Meaning* by Victor Frankl. It was a time in my life when I was trying to make existential meaning out of what seemed like a lot of craziness at home and in the world. This best-selling classic book chronicles Frankl's experiences as an Auschwitz concentration camp inmate during WWII, where he found, even in the most terrible of situations, that a person still has the freedom to choose how they respond to their circumstances.

For Frankl, it wasn't so much about finding out the "meaning of life," but about continually giving meaning to what is given to us. His life did not begin again once he was released from the concentration camp. He was not waiting to live his best possible life until the moment when the war was over and he walked out of the prison. He was alive, loving, full, present, generous, and compassionate while he was behind bars. His family had been murdered, he was living in a cell, but he still had an open heart, reaching out to others to share even the last piece of his precious stale bread.

Can we be as brave and compassionate during our journey? Can we, even in the midst of our own pain and story, be present enough to give meaning to the moment-to-moment experience of our life, and move from a place of love and gratitude? Certainly that is not always an easy assignment. Yet what good is life if we are in this vast schoolhouse and playground and we don't learn and create meaning from each moment that is given to us? Although my journey has certainly been filled with overwhelming challenges, it has also been woven together with overwhelming acts of kindness, generosity, friendship, and love to create the intricate and beautiful tapestry of my life right now.

Thankfully, I'm not waiting for my life to "begin again." It never stopped. This journey is my life. Every beautiful, crazy, up, down, all around, and "take what you get" moment of it. I don't want to miss any of it while I'm waiting.

The journey is everything. The journey is right here, right now.

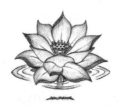

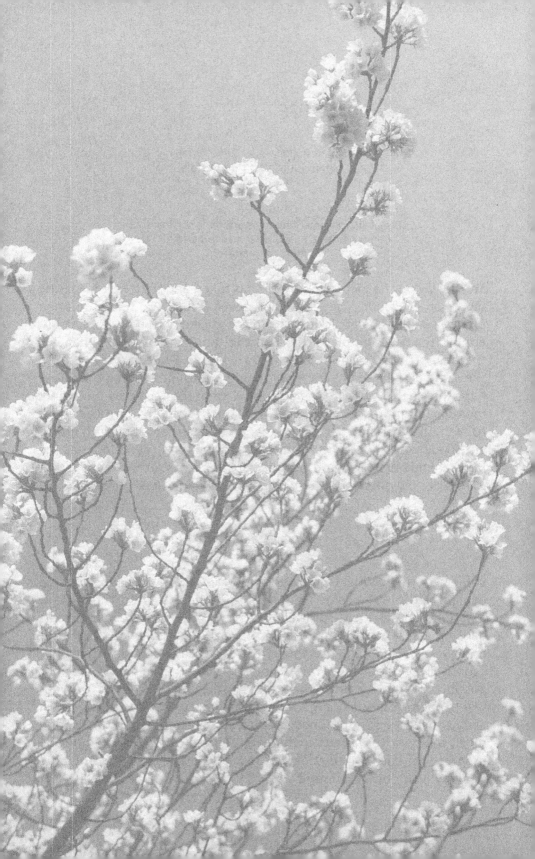

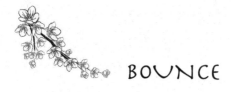

# BOUNCE

Our greatest glory is not in never falling,
but in rising every time we fall.
-Confucious

Resilience:
The ability of something to return to its original shape
after it has been pulled, stretched, pressed, or bent.
-Merriam-Webster

The jigsaw puzzle picture of my life has fallen and shattered into little pieces on the floor. The pieces will never connect to form the same picture again. I slowly pick up each piece, mixed with new pieces gathered in the fall, and place them on the table one by one. What will the new picture reveal? Many might want to feverishly try to form the same picture again, cramming sharp edges into curved ones. Perhaps that is the meaning of suffering. I embrace each new piece and, moment by moment, allow the unfolding. A new picture continues to form. It's a somewhat familiar landscape perhaps, but with different shading and overtones. Something in the foreground fades as the background bursts forward. Sections are gone altogether. Empty spaces reflect new gifts and adventures yet to be revealed.

Some have asked what is the most important quality to have along the healing path. Many come to mind, but perhaps the most important is "bounce." A resilient spirit allows us to continually rebound, reorganize, reboot, and recalibrate with every new challenge. Resiliency is flow and the endless opportunity to create a new direction. We cannot prepare ourselves for all possible outcomes in life. We cannot possibly foresee our future needs and anticipate how, when, or what will happen—especially on our healing journey. We do know we will always need to stay grounded, centered, peaceful, courageous, and meet, moment to moment, whatever comes our way. I could not be prepared for each moment on this journey. However, I was prepared to allow it to flow and unfold.

As resilient warriors going through diagnosis and treatment, we are asked to free-fall into each new twist and turn. We tolerate high levels of ambiguity. We focus on what we can do versus what we can't. We learn to both laugh and cry as our hair falls out in clumps, or our stomach turns in nausea, as if perpetually stalled at the top of a huge ferris wheel. We learn from our experience and are not bitter. We become flexible like bamboo, bending with the winds of constant change during our journey. We are alchemists. We are made stronger by the fire as we turn the coal of our challenges into a shining diamond of resiliency. Embracing resiliency during our healing path turns a series of potentially traumatic events in our lives into a schoolhouse of learning and transformation. Seemingly adverse events unfold. We enter the diagnosis, assessment, and staging. Our ability to cope is challenged with treatment. We face a "new normal" as we seek to make adjustments to living with shifts in our physical and emotional realities. There are so many opportunities along this path to flex and strengthen our resiliency muscle. We are continually asked to find wonder, joy, grace, and beauty along the way. To laugh. To love. To be grateful to be alive. To bounce.

A resilient spirit doesn't limit itself to what it thinks it knows, but to the mystery, awe, and wonder of life. We embrace ambiguity and ask ourselves what can we learn from our journey. Patience? Letting go? An open heart? Courage? Humility? Inner peace? Gratitude?

In the beautiful art of aikido, which is taught at our dojo, students endlessly practice ukemi: falling and rolling. The student blends with the incoming energy, rolls with seeming effortlessness to the ground, then rises to a stance of center and calm. First, the fall and roll is a thud, a circle filled with square edges and the sound of fear. It takes thousands of repetitions to work off the hard edges and be able to smoothly "bounce" back to their feet. It has been said that we learn to fall so we can learn to pick ourselves back up. Resiliency is the ultimate act of freedom that allows us to stay open and transform each challenge into wisdom, harmony, and new opportunity. Our healing journeys and life itself are our constant practice in being able to bounce in the face of whatever comes our way. A resilient spirit strengthens our resourcefulness and creativity, and also sustains us in our challenges. Resiliency gives birth to more resiliency. We become warriors who continue to walk with courage and openness through our human experience, no matter what the challenge. We reside in a trust of the 360° perspective of our life.

Toddlers are my teachers. Learning how to walk, they fall, smile, laugh, then with wobbling legs, attempt to stand up once again only to fall. Eager to try again and again, they finally walk, run, and soar. We are also toddlers, learning to walk among the challenges of being human, falling time after time. We tend to fear the fall and don't usually rise with a smile and a chuckle. However, falling is our salvation. Resiliency is the act of getting up. It doesn't matter if we fall down. Falling is our opportunity to rise upward again and again. Falling down is part of the bounce. If we never fall, we don't learn resiliency and how to recover from the skinned knees of our emotional and physical injuries. Each fall is not a permanent landing on the ground, but a springboard that creates stronger legs to push ourselves upward time and time again. If we try to prepare for each fall, we get caught up in fear and worry. We freeze movement. During our healing journey, we need to become experts at free-fall and rising again and again. We must gather every last ounce of strength and fortitude to return day in and day out to the regime of treatment, a changing body, difficult decisions, not knowing, or too much knowing. If we trust that we have what it takes to always rise again, then we can free-fall into wherever the present moment takes us.

Resiliency means that we don't give power and drama to our situation by telling our story of "woe is me" over and over again. This only holds us to the past and "freezes" our experience. Like a phonograph record stuck, we then continue to repeat what was instead of what is moment to moment. As resilient warriors, we trust the awareness that everything is going to be all right, because all right doesn't depend upon the state of our body, but upon the voice of our soul.

Graced with the opportunity of learning to overcome challenges of all kinds, we bounce back stronger, wiser, and more personally powerful. Then all of life's inevitable difficulties are met with buoyancy and grace.

Resiliency can shine in a situation as seemingly small as the grace we give to the nurse who has to search for our vein to insert the IV needle, and as large as giving thanks to the whole experience of our healing journey. It is in getting in the car, time and time again, for the next treatment. It is in rising to each new day and appreciating all our blessings. It is accepting whatever is, moment to moment.

The serenity prayer used by those struggling with addiction is especially poignant as we travel through our journey. It could be renamed the "resiliency prayer" as we reach out to a higher power to grant us the serenity to accept the things we cannot change, the courage to change the things we can, and the wisdom to know the difference. Our resiliency springs forth from the great freedom we have to always be able to control how we respond to any situation, whether it's the waiting, the side effects, the not knowing, the emotional and physical challenges, or what we can no longer do.

Resiliency doesn't mean that we find it easy to deal with difficulty, nor does it mean we never feel angry, sad, or worried during the tough times. It does mean that we aren't overwhelmed by each wave crashing on our shore. We see the big picture. We find the positive as we learn from our path. We let our circumstances become our teacher and ask: "What can I learn from this?" We allow people to help us. We accept our experience, reflect on our feelings, expect things to work out, and realize that we can't change what happens, but we can change how we respond to it. We walk through our experience trusting the journey.

I was chatting with a friend and she said, "You have really been pushing the envelope." After she left, I did a Google search on this phrase. I knew the spirit of the words, but didn't know from whence they sprang. The words come from aviation and testing the technical limits of a plane's performance by pushing its envelope of safety.

Yes, I pondered, her words were true. Not the kind of pushing that tires the body and so often can slow healing. Instead, the kind that, while respecting limits, also tests them so I can continue to create a larger and larger envelope of healing. I have been perpetually pushing the envelope since my surgery (perhaps in life in general) by turning my head a bit further, lifting a paper cup with a little more water weight, walking a few more steps, slicing a vegetable, and cutting pieces of my art materials. Her words made me wonder where I would be now if I hadn't been pushing the envelope from the moment after my surgery.

Whether it is in healing or the ins and outs of our lives, we never really know until we try. We create our own envelope, and sometimes we even lick it closed. We often complain about the box we find ourselves in, forgetting that we are the ones who set the perimeters, and so continually have the choice to expand them. We decide what elements of our experience to push or not push. Conscious efforts let us know to either respect or expand the limits. Every day is a new day full of choices, new discoveries, expanding boundaries, or nothing at all. Each day and each moment is an opportunity to experience our resiliency.

The sky is the limit! No matter what our life circumstance, we can always venture off our little acre of security for a more expansive landscape. Here's to pushing our envelopes and not accepting predictions or limitations from anyone! Bounce!

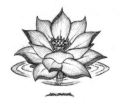

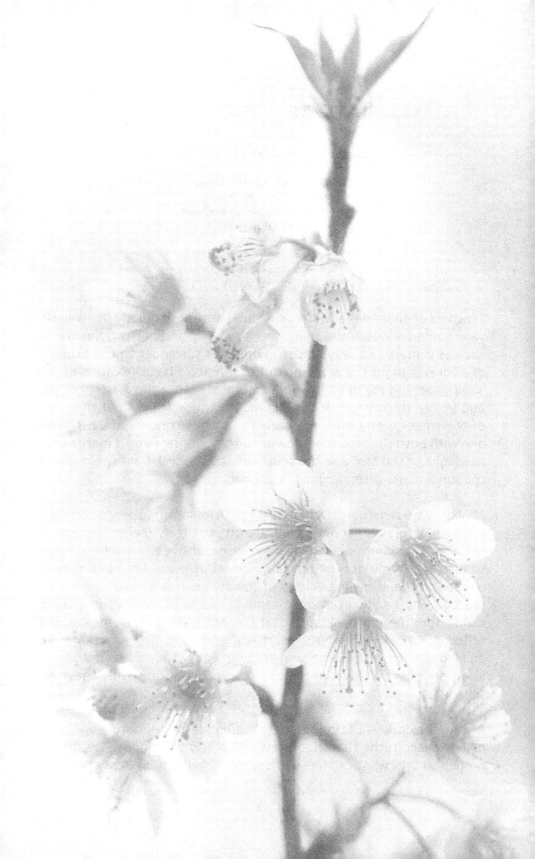

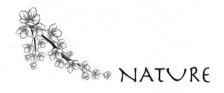

# NATVRE

Adapt the pace of nature...her gift is patience.

Like a crocus in the snow,
I stand knee-deep in Winter
Holding Springtime in my heart.
-Joan Walsh Anglund

Nature is the one place where miracles not only happen,
but they happen all the time.
-Thomas Wolfe

Teachers of all shapes and sizes surround me as I sit quietly in my back-yard garden. I watch the snail, ever so slowly and patiently, carry its shell as it makes its way across my patio. I surrender to the expanse of a forever night sky reaching out to infinity. I feel the caress of the wind wrapping me in its invisible embrace. I sense the majesty of the bud before the miracle of the bloom. The invisible depth of the roots of the trees quietly offer me their strength. Sitting in stillness, I am one with both the blooming flower and the wilting petal. I merge with the flight of the bird and the scurry of the squirrel. I am the rising of the sun and its surrender into the horizon.

My backyard sanctuary surrounds me with its soothing peace each day. I've always felt very connected to nature, but truly feel at home with her now. I am continually healed by her expansive sky, stillness, space to just "be," reminders of renewal and rebirth, and her embodiment of the spiritual, timeless energy of the divine. It is a most welcoming space for my slowly returning morning practice of meditation, prayer, caring for the plants, adapted tai chi and qigong movements, and reflection. Flocks of finches, sparrows, and doves joyfully flutter to and fro as they feed, bathe, and enjoy the day. They all seem to trust in my stillness and love. In the silence, we join as one. Only the mind separates.

During the darkest of times, the unfolding seasons of nature will offer us her deep truths that give perspective and offer hope. Treatment propels us into what can feel like a perpetual winter. She covers everything with a protective layer of snow, but teaches us that underneath, all is very much alive, although dormant. The dark winter of our discontent may be long, stormy, and barren. However it is followed by the bloom and joy of spring that melts away the darkness with its light, warmth, and rebirth. All is reborn as the crocus keeps moving towards the light and breaks through the hard protective ground to bloom. So too shall we. Torrents of spring rain are then followed by the warm and long days of summer. Amid the seeming constriction of our treatment, summer gives us her expansive spirit, wild abandon, and sense of freedom. Autumn asks us to drop what is no longer essential as her leaves fall to the ground as she gathers nourishment from deep within her roots. Our energy drops deep into our cells to heal.

We go through treatment, but life continues to unfold with all its wonder and awe. The vast ocean tide rises and ebbs in an endless cycle. We are a part of this infinite rhythm of life. Yes, there is decay and seeming death, but also an endless cycle of rejuvenation and renewal. Nature reminds us that nothing is permanent and that time stops for no one. The Earth rotates around the sun. The sun sets only to rise anew the next day. Clouds appear and can quickly drift away. There are times of light and warmth, cold and darkness, growth and expansion, and surrendering and letting go to receive new gifts and growth. If we open to the lessons of nature, we feel her nurturing pulse of life. We experience no death, but a flow of ever-changing forms.

When we sit quietly in nature, we are invited to experience the wonderment of existence with all our senses, freeing our mind to embrace the present moment. With our mind and body moving into stillness, we naturally slip into greater balance and healing. We shift our attention beyond our small, physical existence, beyond our pain, and beyond our own challenges and circumstances to recognize that we are inextricably connected to the wonder, awe, and miracle of the universe. Nature can be our therapist on our journey, offering an ever-present source of solace and stillness to listen to our fears and embrace our tears. If we allow her, she will be our unfailing, comforting companion and honored teacher throughout our journey of recovery.

Let each season in nature, and within our healing, surrender to the next. Let us embrace whatever season we are in, accepting and aligning with its energy and influence. If we can find the meaning within each season, we can trust that our treatment is also a cycle with a definite purpose. We then know that whatever our current season, this too shall pass. Everything changes.

## SUMMER

The long summer days stretch out their arms, embracing me with warmth and comfort, permeating me with that feeling of endless youth. Yet this is definitely a different kind of summer for me. It is a summer of grace, love, healing, and patience. I look at my garden and see a statue of the meditative Buddha, who said that "the greatest prayer is patience." The Bible says, "To everything there is a season, and a time and purpose to everything under heaven." This is my time to heal. This is my season and, as with all seasons, its cycle and rhythm will carry me on to the next. Summer's early morning heat invites me into its warm and loving embrace. As day turns to dusk, children's voices echo off the pavement as they steal the last moments of sunset before being called to their homes. I am at once a child of ten playing outside as the curtain of dusk falls while ignoring my mother's call to come home, and an adult limited in movement as I sit in healing stillness.

Unleashed freedom and boundless energy were always my unfailing companions within the heat of summer. Now I sit in healing stillness in my patio chair and watch green leaves, colorful blooms, and the blue blanket of the sky.

Summer was once a time of riding the surf, but now I'm riding waves of nausea from the chemotherapy. Soaking in the soothing rays of the sun while lying on my beach towel is now soaking in the radiation waves while lying on the conveyor belt. Putting my mask on and going snorkeling is now being bolted into my big neon green mask and going for a ride in the radiation tunnel. Late summer evenings outside hiking in the Whittier Hills are now late summer evenings sitting in stillness in my patio chair, listening to the last song of the chirping birds before snuggling under the sheets.

Perhaps the outside props and circumstances of my life differ, but inside I remain the same. I am grateful for all I have, living moment to moment, loving, laughing, and letting life move through me. Summer, always and once again, welcomes me into her warm embrace.

# FALL

I watch the golden leaves fall willingly and lightheartedly from the two poplar trees in my yard. The leaves sway playfully in the wind, performing a final last dance before hitting the ground. Some stop to rest on my lap and shoulders. It is their time to let go. What if these leaves hung tight and resisted change as we often do? It is so easy to hold on to what was instead of letting go. So easy to default to the familiar instead of embracing the unknown. If only we could shed what is no longer needed with such grace and beauty. These leaves protected me from the blistering rays of the summer sun. Now their descent creates barren branches that invite sunshine to warm me from the now crisp chill of fall. They stand barren, naked, vulnerable, open, yet strong. Change happens, yet all remains perfect. I give thanks to all the trees for their great lessons of letting go to allow for new birth, new opportunities, and the advent of spring.

After my surgery, a friend planted sunflower seeds in my backyard. Now the sprouts form a welcoming flower facing upward toward the sun. The miracle of the bloom and the miracle of my healing are one, and they meet in a joyous dance of renewal and rebirth.

Fall leads us to a balance of darkness and light. At autumn's equinox, day and night are of equal length. Days slowly get shorter and darkness comes to visit earlier and earlier. We begin to pull inward and find ourselves curling up like a cat in our own heat. We learn to befriend the darkness as a place of stillness and silence. It is a place that beckons us to rest and allow space for our healing. The bare branches outside remind us again that everything changes. We also learn to trust that the bud and blossom may be disappearing into the advent of winter, but that all will lead to rebirth in the upcoming spring.

## WINTER

I sit in my patio chair and once again gaze outward to my backyard sanctuary. This small plot of rented land has been my comfort, my teacher, and my healer. Nature gracefully and easily has unfolded alongside me with each new cycle of my healing. Winter, with its longer periods of darkness, now asks for even deeper reflection, silence, and contemplation. Nature always gives me an open invitation to quiet my mind, still my soul, and hear my inner voice and truth. What better friend can one have? All I need to do is be still and she constant-ly reminds me that all is eternal, life is an endless cycle, and that we are all one with everything.

What if we could see the true meaning and value of the "winters" of our lives? What if we could recognize their necessity for new life and possibilities for renewal? What if we could surrender to the knowledge that all will reappear in our upcoming spring? What if we embraced the barren landscape of our "winter" as a time of healing hibernation that connects deeply with our own being, and so to the infinite source that connects us all? Winter asks me to trust, let go, and surrender. It beckons me to feel the abiding light inside within its darkness. It reminds me that everything is under its protective cover, being nour-ished to rise again. When we are deep in the winter of our recovery, our energies have gone inward to deeply heal us and will eventually expand outward into new, vibrant life.

## SPRING

The patio chair that I sat in during months of quiet healing is now faded and worn through use and the unfolding seasons. It tells a story of stillness, patience, and healing. Cushions are flattened and stained with dropped food that never made its way into my mouth's tiny pin-hole opening. A glance at it triggers memories of sitting with both arms gently resting on pillows propped at its sides, minimal move-ment, breathing ever so slowly in discomfort and pain, gazing at my garden out of one blurred eye, one arm in a sling and the other only able to pick up a paper cup, and of a TV tray placed in front of me to eat and to look at cards from Team Suzette. This simple green chair is saturated with moment-to-moment, breath-to-breath living from summer to now spring. With the advent of this season of rebirth, I purchase a new patio chair, along with a portable outside desk for sketching and writing.

Spring is a time for cleaning out and making way for fresh possibilities and new growth. It is a time to begin again. Rebirth and renewal are everywhere. Colors explode, leaves return, shades of green paint the landscape, rain washes everything fresh, and the hardness of the ground softens to beckon new life to push through toward the sun. Hesitant buds in my garden are risking bloom into the light of the day.

With each new glance, it seems that the green, chi-filled trees grow fuller with leaves to provide shade from the sun. What was within now shows itself without. All rises toward the sun's warmth, and so do I.

Let the warmth of spring and its healing energy of new beginnings saturate every cell. With the longer and lighter days of spring, what once seemed impossible now feels hopeful. Inside, we remember that the energy of spring is always there to wake, nurture, and revitalize. Hope blossoms. Joy explodes. Our spirits soar with the miracle of new birth.

## A BOW TO MY HEALING TEACHERS

### The Sky

The sky is covered in dark and daunting storm clouds, but I find a sliver of blue. When I can't find the sliver of blue, I hold on to my memory of the blue sky that always resides underneath, not unlike moving toward the remembrance of the light. The sky is forever, as is our soul. We are the sky. Clouds, like the constant flicker of our thoughts and the circumstances of our life, are just the ever-changing parade passing through at the mercy of the wind and sun. Treatment, or whatever our challenge, will eventually pass like the clouds to reveal the endless blue sky.

### The Birds

I listen to the melody of the birds, really listen, as if I have paid hundreds of dollars for a backyard seat this close to the orchestra pit at the symphony. I hear each individual sound as well as its magnificent blending into the chorus. Each rat-a-tat, each chirp, every squeal, and an occasional whistle is like a myriad of instruments all joining together for a soulful melody. I hear where one rests and the other begins. I hear the trumpet and the saxophone, along with the percussion and shrill flute. It is one magnificent orchestra. I need only be still and listen. I hear their joy in each moment. Carefree. Vibrant. Alive. How blessed we are if only we could be still enough to listen.

## The Flowers

Each flower I see reflects back to me the importance of opening my heart to the world. The bud risks the bloom, then embraces both the torrents of rain and the warmth of the sun. The whipping wind can cause its petals to fly, but the caress of a gentle breeze soothes. We want to shut out so much on our journey, but how much do we miss? A closed heart receives nothing, but the risk of opening it allows us to blossom and embrace everything. If we still ourselves and gaze into the eye of the flower, we will see the intricacy of their veins, the multitude of colors that look solid at first glance, and the delicacy of its petals. Each one is different as it reaches toward the sun. Each of us is different, with our special gifts to give and divine purpose.

## The Trees

The trees are forever humble with their deep, hidden strength. Roots that sink deep into the earth stabilize and ground them. They need not announce their power, for it is felt in each branch and leaf. Their lives are long and often impervious to the elements. They reach out to all as a home and a shelter. They deserve great praise and glory for their beauty. The trees teach us strength, inner peace, healing, and the power and center found from deep stillness and being rooted to the earth.

## The Water

Even if it is only the sound of a fountain, water can remind us to soften and flow around obstacles. There is no need to meet anything in a head-on collision, especially diagnosis and recovery. If we are open, the sound of water can wash away our concerns, continually reminding us to let go. Nothing in life is permanent and fixed. If we soften, then everything empties and expands into open space. Water meets challenges by moving around them and changing its shape while never stopping its natural flow. Its constant, free-flowing, gentle force polishes the edges of the roughest stone. Let us find the flow within us that gives us the strength of water's gentle yet powerful nature. Let our emotions, our circumstances, and our challenges be fluid and resilient. If we resist, if we say no instead of yes, everything will stagnate and form a cesspool. Let water soothe and purify us, whether it be our garden sprinklers, our small dining room fountain, a nightly bath, a gentle rain, or the roar of the ocean. All can be our gentle reminders to relax, surrender, and let go.

## The Wind

I sat for countless hours watching the waving of the leaves from the invisible breath and breeze of the wind. The wind is the ultimate magician, with its sleight of hand and invisible tricks. It can be as tame, comforting, and soothing as a summer breeze, or as strong, forceful, and destructive as a fierce tornado. The wind reminds us of our thoughts, which are also powerful and create great calm or great turmoil with a seemingly invisible presence.

The wind asks us to move with it or feel great resistance. On a hot air balloon ride many years ago, a rider in the basket with me lit up a cigarette. I was amazed that the match did not blow out with the strong wind that swept us through the clouds. The pilot said it was because we were moving with, not against, the wind. How often in life do we resist where the winds of change are blowing us, instead of allowing them to take us where they will with great trust and abandon? The only constant in life is change. The wind reminds us to let go and enjoy the ride.

The wind and the air are one. The wind is nothing but air in motion. The air always surrounds and sustains us, but is often taken for granted. Air, not unlike our connection to spirit, is ever-present. The air is our lifeline and so we must remember to breathe deeply into the depths of each cell. Each breath of air is our healing.

## Animals

Animals may have a more simple existence than us and yet the spiritual goals we often hope to attain come as easily to them as breathing. They are masters of living in the present moment and offer us unconditional love. Animals have true beauty. They don't need mirrors, weight loss programs, or self-help books. They find joy in simple pleasures. Patience and forgiveness are their gifts to us. They lift our spirits in their sense of play and unleashed joy. Look to them for how to move through illness, or throughout the day. They are in no rush, rest in perfect stillness, and move in natural spontaneity. For them, time has no meaning. The squirrels bury their nuts, the birds flutter to and fro, and dogs lick our faces with thoughtless abandon. They are free from assumption, judgment, and comparison. A bird is not trying to act like a squirrel, nor is it saying that it's more beautiful or greater than a tree. They do not lament about how they suffer more because the wind is more challenging at their back or the sun is more harsh on their skin. They reflect the perfect consciousness of the beauty of who they are without consideration and thought. Finches arrive in great number and eat slowly in their shared community, without chasing each other away. When finished, they take great joy in soaring flight. The squirrels are full of natural whimsy, play, and perky expression. Dogs and cats love without fear to find a place deep in our heart. Each animal is an integral part of nature, offering us lessons on how to simply be, as well as how to heal. Embrace them.

When I asked the infinite for peace and comfort, the answer was: "I am here, comforting you in the chirp of every bird, in every blade of grass, every bloom, and the individual leaf on every tree. I am the flutter of every bird's wing, the endless palette of colors in the universe, the embrace of the wind, and each vein of a flower's petals. I am in the rise of the morning sun, the light of the full moon, and the darkness of the eclipse. I am in the tiniest ant making its way across the patio, and each root reaching out to unimpeded distances. I am the divine artistry unfolding with an invisible paintbrush in each ever-changing cloud, falling leaf, star in the sky, dance of the shadows, and still, timeless second. I am the power, the expansiveness, and the love in each pulse of life that surrounds you and joins us all together. I am wherever you look. Within you and without. We are one."

During the dark and difficult time of diagnosis and treatment, if we can surround ourselves with the magnificent, loving, and healing power of nature, then it will guide us to become aware of our own remarkable inner forces that allow us to persevere through the darkest of times. The stillness and quiet of nature may then lead us to greater clarity and insight. If we reach out in emptiness, listen in silence, and leave our wild minds at the doorstep, we will learn deep and abiding lessons from her endless beauty. Nature will not only comfort us, but lead us gently and compassionately to our own true essence.

Allow nature to be your great teacher. Remember that fall never tries to resist the coming of winter. Spring doesn't complain that summer is coming once again. Let each season in nature, and our healing, surrender to the next. Nature is very skilled at accepting the "what is" and using it to unfold into the "what can be." So must we. Make time for yourself every day to rest in nature. Walk barefoot on the grass. If you don't have the energy to walk, stand, or sit. Truly listen to the chirping of the birds. Cuddle with a pet. Smell a flower. Experience nature's peace deep in your center. Let time become meaningless in the inhale of a rose, the gaze at an expansive blue sky, a breeze on your face, and within the hidden strength of a tree. Accept the gifts of nature, and embrace her healing energy with immense gratitude and an open heart.

We are all involved in this great dance of life. The blossom, the chirp of each bird, the afternoon shadow, and the soft illumination of a crescent moon are at one with us. We must always let our souls and hearts be wide open to the healing gifts of nature. Each day, let us give great gratitude for the miracle of life that surrounds us. Let the magnificence of nature be your soothing, patient, timeless, colorful, constant, and ever-changing companion on your healing journey.

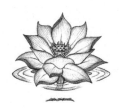

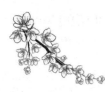

# CHANGE THE LYRICS

Words at the end of a phone. A doctor gives me the results of my biopsy and the diagnosis. Past images flash of my dad, my mom, and my boyfriend/best friend, all gone from cancer. Then I fast-forward to the possible clips of a similar sad fate. Finally, there is a crash landing in the present moment of my diagnosis. In January 2013, a phone call said I had stage three lymphoma. Another one in April 2014 said that I had stage four metastasized squameous cell cancer. With each call, the Scrabble board of my life changed. Words like incurable, metastasis, surgery, chemotherapy, radiation, advanced, and aggressive appeared. However, I have added my own words, such as miracles, milestones, cured, healed, love, gratitude, and amazing. Words have power, and cancer carries a heavy weight. So I have changed the vocabulary and the Scrabble board in front of me to words that uplift, strengthen, and heal. For those of you who play Scrabble, I have used them all on the triple word score.

An oncologist I saw once said to me, "After treatment is over, we have to be concerned about reoccurrence and continued metastasis." My thought: "How about we concern ourselves with total remission and miracles?"

There are no problems, only challenges.

I used to visit the nursing home to see my aunt. Her roommate was a very wise woman struggling with many ailments. One day, I was there and saw that she was hooked up to tubes, confined to bed, and barely able to visit. She told me what had happened and then added, "Not to worry. To be like this is just my assignment for right now." What a wonderful way to look at challenges. We are all given our assignments, some seemingly more difficult than others, throughout our lives. She truly knew how to change the lyrics.

We need to get rid of the gavel. We travel through life holding it in our hand and striking it with a definitive crack on the hardwood of our experience. GOOD! BAD! Then we organize our circumstances, as obsessive bean counters, into tiny bins of yes and no, right and wrong. Wisdom is often disguised by our judgments and so possible kernels of clarity and truth get suffocated by our false thinking. However, if we let go of the hard shell of judgment and resistance, accepting each experience as a lesson to be learned, we can be transformed.

My grandma would make her favorite stew by mixing together whatever ingredients were in the refrigerator. I would say to myself: "Yuck! I don't even like onions! Yikes, what is that green thing she is cutting up? Oh no! Is that red vegetable a beet? No way! Oh yum, corn!" I sat in definitive judgment as each item was dropped into the boiling pot of water. However, somehow the simmering mix of ingredients created an aroma that would beckon me closer and closer. The first sip would have me begging for more of "Gertie's Goo."

Each experience creates the other. Who are we to determine what is good and bad? We can't see the 360° picture. We can't separate and define each experience. It is the threads of all colors that create the intricate, beautiful tapestry of our lives. We need to bow to whatever is happening without judgment. Everything is a sacred gift and lesson. We can then learn to appreciate the "Gertie's Goo" that is our lives.

It is hard and constant training to put aside the gavel strike of good and bad and to say yes to our path without judgment. This is especially true during our diagnosis and recovery. Changing the lyrics allows us to move from no to yes, continually bowing to all as our teacher. A day in our lives is made not by circumstances deemed good or bad, but by our lyrics and connection to all whose path we cross.

## Changing the Lyrics

Saying no: It can't be.
Saying yes: It is.

Saying no: This sucks.
Saying yes: Lessons await.

Saying no: Why me?
Saying yes: Why not me?

Saying no: My dad died of cancer.
Saying yes: I will heal.

Saying no: How long will I live?
Saying yes: I have the gift of life each day.

Saying no: It isn't fair.
Saying yes: This is an unfolding gift.

Saying no: The door to my heart slams shut.
Saying yes: The door to my heart opens to let in light, love, and healing.

Saying no: I don't want to feel.
Saying yes: I want to experience it all.

Saying no: I tighten and contract.
Saying yes: My body opens and relaxes.

Saying no: This pain will never go away.
Saying yes: Everything changes.

Saying no: I want this to be over.
Saying yes: The journey is everything.

Saying no: I'm scared.
Saying yes: I trust the journey.

Saying no: No one could understand.
Saying yes: Everybody cares.

Saying no: Everyone thinks they know what is best for me.
Saying yes: Everyone loves me.

Saying no: I fret about what will be.
Saying yes: I rest in what is.

Saying no: People want to save me with their particular religion.
Saying yes: They want for me what has brought them comfort.

Saying no: I am my illness.
Saying yes: I am an infinite soul.

Saying no: I feel all alone.
Saying yes: Separation is an illusion.

Saying no: I feel like I am going to die.
Saying yes: I am the miracle of life!

Saying no: This will never end.
Saying yes: It is just this moment.

Saying no: I am in horrible pain.
Saying yes: Everything is an ever-changing sensation.

Saying no: This is miserable.
Saying yes: This is another opportunity to learn and grow.

Saying no: I'll never be the same again.
Saying yes: Life is a continuous flow.

We create the melody of our lives. Do we want it to be a stereophonic funeral dirge in our head, or an inspirational opera? I feel so much better when I change the lyrics. Then my life can become like one of my favorite songs that I can sing along with every day. Uplifting. Opening. Joyful. I am in the car of my life and the windows are open, my hair is blowing, the radio is cranked high, and I sing like no one is listening. When I change the lyrics, I feel my strength, power, and gratitude. It doesn't mean denying the minor chord. A melody can become even more beautiful with a few minor chords that make the sound of the major ones even more inspiring. However, we do not need to live our lives in a minor key.

Some neuroscientists believe we have seventy thousand thoughts a day. If we aren't aware, negative lyrics can create a rut in our mind and we are continually humming a downward tune. These constant thoughts and judgments will close us down and cause us to identify with our pain. This creates more resistance and more suffering.

I went from telling only my family about my initial lymphoma diagnosis to eventually sharing my entire journey with the squameous cell cancer with everyone on the Team Suzette website. This gave me not only the ability to stay in loving connection with everyone during my deep healing, but also the freedom to share my own uplifting lyrics. Then family and friends could sing the same song with me in one joyous chorus. Words of pity, fear, regret, negativity, and apprehension could be overcome with positive lyrics of love, gratitude, and miracles.

There are so many challenges to staying open along the treatment path. So many possibilities to fall into judgment and create negative lyrics. If we are honest, the messages we give ourselves during our treatment are often foreboding and negative. If we went through a day and wrote down all of our thoughts, what would they reveal? Would they be full of fear, worst case scenarios, complaints, and anger? They could possibly sound like the downward lyrics of "These side effects are horrible." "Why me?" "This will never end."

This is how I sought to transform the lyrics during my treatment. "Radiation is so horrible for me and it is destroying my good cells," becomes "Let the rays of radiation find, penetrate, and obliterate all diseased cells, while also proving a protective shield for all my healthy cells, allowing them to grow even stronger."

"It is so painful to have to take off my sling for each radiation treatment," becomes "How sweet is it that the therapist so tenderly helps me ease the sling off my shoulder to put on the gown."

"It hurts to have my face bolted down into the mask and it is so hard to breath," becomes "Ah, there is the compassionate hand of the therapist, gently brushing my hair aside, trying to position each strand so it doesn't pull. She is slowly guiding the hard mesh mask squarely on my face so it is most comfortable for me. My face is like clay that softens and conforms inside the mask."

"I feel all alone in this tunnel. It is dark, suffocating, scary, confining, and never-ending," becomes "Ah, there is the therapist's loving voice guiding me into the tunnel and periodically reassuring me during the ride. My breath relaxes, comforts, and opens me. Soon I will be out of the tunnel and the compassionate hand of the therapist will give me a gentle, loving back rub as I sit up."

"Chemotherapy is horrible. It makes me so sick and poisons me with endless side effects," becomes "The fluid is penetrating deeply to remove all unwanted critters and heal me forevermore."

"How much longer will this go on? I want to get on with my life!" becomes "What is this teaching me about life? About my life?"

We are the script writers, directors, choreographers, and main characters in the play of our lives. Changing our lyrics means letting go of "our old story." It is changing the words we tuck ourselves into bed with each night, play first thing in the morning, and repeat endlessly throughout our day. The stories we tell ourselves influence each breath, feeling, mood, and action. It is not healing for us to live with an old script. It is as if we put on a jacket because we are cold, but once warmer, we keep telling the story of how cold we are. We need to be right here, right now. We do not say, "Oh, yesterday I felt so awful,"

and relay the story of those aches and pains even though today we feel slightly better. We must continue to sing out each circumstance we are given as a gift to help us grow spiritually. Our story must embrace the bigger picture and the faith that all will unfold with great love, knowing, peace, and purpose. My body would feel so much better each time I gave light to a positive change, however slight. "I am able to keep a little more food down the hatch." Or "I slept a little longer through the night," even if "a little longer" was only five minutes.

We especially need to change the lyrics to the story of the big "C." The word carries so much power. Those going through treatment will say, "I have stage three cancer," as if it is something defined, solid, concrete, irremovable, and their identity. Everyone quivers and draws their energy inward when they hear the news. It is all too easy to let this label define our journey. Then we become the looming, dark, foreboding shadow that is this word. We are defined by everyone's fears and experiences of their own journey and that of their loved ones. I rarely used the word. It confined and robbed me of my identity as a beam of radiant light beneath the ever-changing realities of my body. For what is cancer but a group of cells gone bad? It is not who we are. I changed the lyrics to "My body is out of balance," "I have some unwelcome cells," "I have been diagnosed with," and not "I have." It is not something we own, nor does it hold us hostage. It is but a set of fluctuating symptoms and cellular changes. Cancer is merely a diagnosis, because at any moment we are healed. Changing the lyrics means to keep moving toward the light. Each word can become a prayer or added weight to a sinking ship. I feel so much better when I sing along to uplifting lyrics rather than a depressing tune.

No matter what your circumstance, create your own uplifting lyrics, sing to your most inspiring song, dance if only in your imagination, crank open the door to your heart, and express your joy as if no one is listening. Change your lyrics and change your life.

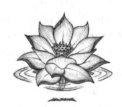

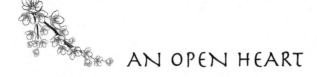

# AN OPEN HEART

The best and most beautiful things in the world cannot be seen
or even heard, but must be felt with the heart.
-Helen Keller

The greatest gift you'll ever learn
is just to love, and be loved in return.
-Nat King Cole, "Nature Boy"

The way is not in the sky.
The way is in the heart
-Buddha

Blessed are the pure in heart, for they shall see God.
-Matthew 5:8

I had been writing update after update, but hadn't ventured backward in time to revisit them. Six months after my surgery, I didn't reread them, but instead rewound the movie projector to the first message from intensive care, then fast-forwarded back to the present moment. I was met with a kaleidoscope of fragmented moments in time frozen by my words, pictures, and feelings. Baby steps turned into leaps, challenges into triumphs, and reflections into releases. Mostly, I was somewhat overcome by how much I had opened my heart, without hesitation and with abandon, as I wrote to everyone. Any walls I might have had were shattered by the explosion of insults to my body, the slowing down, the trust and surrender to whatever was happening, receiving all the love and generosity of Team Suzette, and continually living moment to moment.

Glancing through these updates, I felt a bit naked. I wrote them each month to allow the rhythm and pulse of my life to reach out to everyone while I was restricted in movement and in deep healing. It brought me great joy to express my immense gratitude and love to everyone when I wasn't able to do it in person. In them, any armor was discarded and my heart was flung wide open. Being so open can be a scary and vulnerable place, exposed and perhaps judged. However, it seems to me that my journey here on this planet has been to be increasingly stripped to the core, to reside in and share who I truly am. The best I can do is always try to honor the truth as I experience it. If I let any masks down, trust life, embrace love, open my heart, and share without fear, then my spirit can fly and connect more deeply with everything and everyone. So I remain naked, sharing what is real and true for me.

I can't deny the truth that I continue to find in stillness as I move with infinite time, not with the digital clock that can relentlessly press us forward. This slowing down creates stillness. The stillness allows for silence. It is said that silence is the language of God and that everything else is a poor translation. In the stillness and silence through months of recovery, the truth that continued to echo, again and again, is that the essence of our life is to create an unbroken circle of both giving and receiving love. It's funny. I hear myself sounding more and more like one of the sappy greeting cards I often deplore. Yet this continues to be my experience that I can't deny. Who knows? My strange and twisted fate might just be to get a job writing Hallmark love cards!

I will always lean into an open heart and yearn not to break the circle of love that brings us all together. Our journeys are sewn together on the same tapestry of life. We need each other to both give and receive love. What good is being loved if we don't fully open up to receive it, let it saturate every cell, and return it to the world?

Waking up from surgery in intensive care, with the breathing tube and straps on my arms and legs just removed, the reassuring and compassionate face of one of my skillful and empathetic surgeons was an umbrella above me. I held his hand, then tried to draw him closer. The nurse said in a half chuckle, "I think she wants to kiss you." It was true. I pulled him in and rested my lips briefly against his cheek in gratitude for my life, and whispered a loving "thank you."

The oncologists will say, "You really responded well to the chemotherapy and radiation." Others will say, "That fourteen-hour surgery was amazing." Some will reflect: "Prayers and positive thoughts have healed you." Others jokingly say that all those organic green veggie drinks didn't give those suckers half a chance. Some feel that "keeping relaxed in a healing, meditative state" was the key. However, what is it that ultimately heals? My experience is that love is the healing force, allowing us to deeply receive all the treatments, prayers, and positive thoughts. Love is the brilliant, golden thread that weaves everything together and makes all things possible. Everyone's love continued to keep me open. When in the closed-curtained, deep, and dark of the night, when my nerves would fire with wild abandon, head unable to turn, and muscles twist in pain, anxiety could appear like an unwelcome visitor. When alone, longing for a hand to hold but finding none, contracting in fear would be like turning the key to lock the prison door behind me. However, time and time again, when caught in the seemingly solitary confinement of symptoms from surgery and treatment, what would save me was opening up to receive the flood of love and kindness from everyone, and in turn, to send love out. Opening up and connecting to everything and everyone created the space to minimize my pain by wrapping me in a huge blanket of love, peace, and connection.

It is not just the love we receive that heals, but the love we give. It is the endless circle that knows no separation. Love is the essence of life, no matter our circumstances. Staying open and connecting to a power much greater than our small self allows miracles to flow freely and with immense grace. You cannot possibly give nor receive too much love during any journey. When in doubt, open up to love and gratitude. The love we give to others connects us with the tsunami of universal love. We are each important drops in the endless ocean of love. We need only to be love. Then love naturally flows to us and back to others. The salvation of everyone is truly through deep and abiding love.

Choose love over judgment and fear in each and every unfolding moment.

The open heart allows us to feel the goodness inside and see the world with fresh eyes that notice every small act of kindness. The open heart is our lake with vast and unending width, depth, and breadth that can embrace everything. From the maternity ward to the hospice room, the open heart holds infinity in its pulse. Love whatever is happening? Yes! Say yes to everything? Yes! Love ourselves, love each other, and love the gift of being alive? Yes!

When my heart remained open, I was able to feel the tenderness in each hand-in-hand, heart-to-heart hug. With an open heart, I embraced each loving doorstep delivery, each compassionate, encouraging card, and each guest book message. An open heart allowed me to feel the love each time I was guided in my weakness and impaired vision, the kind spirit of the volunteer escorting me to my first appointment, the thoughtfulness of the gentleman holding the elevator door open, and the sweet sound of the valet remembering my name. Each vegetable bought and chopped by my family, each eye drop positioned into my eye by my sister with love and empathy, and the gift of each jar of homemade organic soup made with the loving hands of my friends embraced me when my heart was open. An open heart allowed the valiant energy of the patients, the commitment, expertise, and graciousness of the doctors, and the empathy of the nurses to inspire and soothe me. My open heart connected me with the heart of infinite love.

We are all here in this journey together. Opening my heart allowed me to stay connected to who I really am rather than a resentful, bitter, and fearful person. I was able to reach out to everyone and connect to the divine. Circumstances don't change who we are. Instead they ask us to be more of what we truly are.

I always have the choice to follow my heart home. An open heart embraces everything from the tiniest ant to the endless blue sky. It softens even the hardest edge of circumstances and receives all like the deepest inhale. The choice is ours. We can allow our hearts to be open doors that swing outward to give and receive love in an endless circle, or we can slam them shut in fear, resentment, and bitterness.

Where am I most at home? My answer used to be that I was at home in my guts. I was at home when my intestines unraveled and opened. I was at home when my raw antenna reached out to take the world's temperature. I was at home in my stomach, which churns when the headlines read "woman raped" or "infant left on the doorstep." I was at home in its dark pit which says "private property" and "no trespassing," but sometimes opened up to meet the world. When the fire burned deep in my belly, red and yellow with the sparks that ignited me, I was at home. When the saxophone cried and the piano keys sang, when the afternoon was still and I took nothing from it, when I would laugh out loud, and when my eyes would moisten, I would return home.

My home has now risen and fills my heart. I reside in its warmth, its glow, its expansiveness, and its connection to everyone and everything. I rest in the always revolving door of the heart where there is no separation between anything or anyone. Every time I say yes, the door to my heart flings open wider, letting more light in, and I come home. I am at home when the gift and glory of each moment is all I need. I am at home in the "I love you," the kind word, the compassionate touch, and the thought-ful gesture. I am at home in my heart when it opens to embrace both the soul on skid row and my next door neighbor blasting his rap music.

I am at home in my heart as it widens into the vast et cetera of open space that says: "Fill me." I'm at home in the palette of blue sky that allows for the shudder of thunder and blaze of lightning, for drips and torrents, and for ominous cloud to both darken and lift. I'm at home in my heart when the stars come out of hiding and their black canvas forgives me of my sins—its million winking eyes are magnificent, even from such a distance.

Love has been the constant throughout every beat of this journey. A love that is free from the passing of seasons and the external circum-stance of any test, treatment, discomfort, and fear. I long to have a permanent residence there. It is the home of insight and intuition, my compass to true north. It is the home of the divine.

No matter what our challenges or circumstances, if during our journey we can allow our minds to drop more fully into our hearts through silence, stillness, and perpetually letting go, then we have come home. We can be love, continuously receiving and giving it without separation in one endlessly flowing circle. Then the healing energy can permeate every cell.

When I was young, math and I weren't the greatest of friends. It didn't seem to have any mystery or mysticism to it. However, I found fractions very compelling as they could be reduced to their common denominator. Our lives are a kaleidoscope of different changing emotions and trajectories, but love remains timeless. It flows outward from inside all of us if we can connect with our heart and the light that illuminates us from within. Different faiths abound, but love joins us as the one common denominator.

Who are we really? Perhaps just another beat, however small, that connects to all beats in our universal, eternal melody. We are one with the prisoner on death row, the saint, the starving child, the newborn baby, and the infinite. The more I can live within my heart now, the closer I am to merging with eternity. My heart has no "disease." The pulse of its beat is the rhythm that dances with the divine as well as each other. The open heart is heaven on earth. The open heart is our healing.

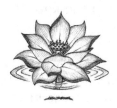

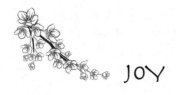

# JOY

Find ecstasy in life;
the mere sense of living is joy enough.
-Emily Dickinson

Joy is prayer; joy is strength:
joy is a net of love by which you can catch souls.
-Mother Theresa

Joy is the simplest form of gratitude.
-Karl Barth

There are many thieves along this journey of treatment that want to steal our joy. Some hold us at gunpoint. Others come in the dark of the night disguised with black masks and rob of us of this most precious and priceless belonging. There is the diagnosis that catches us unaware. Regrets, fears, worries, prognoses, and projections hold us hostage. The drip of chemotherapy, the insult of radiation, the side effects, the not knowing, and the knowing all seek to steal our precious exclamation point.

It is so important to find joy in what is. It is nowhere to be seen if we continue to look at what was. Joy and gratitude are woven together to create the beauty that is our lives, no matter the circumstances.

No one can take our joy away from us. Only we can kidnap it and hold it hostage. Only we can connect to our source of inner joy. Joy does not come to us—we go to it.

Joy sank when I told the "story of my illness", but rose when I expressed the shining light of my spirit.

It left when I fast-forwarded into the future or rewound into the past, but found a home in just one moment at a time.

Joy leapt in my heart each time I thanked the radiation therapist, but took a nosedive when I thought about the next return to the mask.

Joy disappeared when I focused on the pain, but returned when I expanded outward to embrace the discomfort with space and calm.

Joy did a belly flop with each what if, but soared with every what is.

It sank at thoughts of what I couldn't do, but leapt with what I could do.

Pity parties imprisoned my joy, but love set it free.

Joy sat in a dark corner with each regret, but danced at center stage with every soaring hope.

Joy visited with acceptance, but left with resistance and bitterness.

Joy rose up in feeling love, but sank with feeling fear.

Joy came in counting my blessings, but disappeared with counting my misfortunes.

Joy leapt when my heart was open, but tripped and fell to the ground when I shut down.

Joy slammed on its brakes with the thought of the poisons of chemo-therapy, but accelerated with each thought of healing.

Joy appeared when I appreciated my body's hard work to heal, but was banished when I focused on the symptoms and side effects.

Joy softened and caressed the pain, but anger deepened and solidified it.

Joy visited when I waited patiently for my appointment, but left when I sat filled with frustration.

Be joy, and you will find joy.

It is not true that we are robbed of our joy during our diagnosis and treatment. I found joy in the feel of clean sheets and the warm water in the tub on an aching body. Joy visited with the IV needle going in on the first try and during each exit out of the radiation tunnel. Joy flowed through with me with each gentle stroke on my leg from a loved one that soothed the fireworks inside my body. Joy danced when my stitches and drains were removed and when I slipped under the warmth of the heated hospital blankets. Joy came to me with the gift of a beautiful, colorful orchid in full bloom on my dining room table, the sparkle of the white miniature lights strapped around the trees in my backyard, a beautiful handmade quilt for my sterile hospital bed, and the sound of the chimes making music in the breeze. I found it in each flower bursting into bloom and the comfort of the backyard reclining gravity chair on my weakened body. I found joy in my new clothes which zipped up the front as I could no longer pull them over my head. Joy smiled with the final removal of my sling and pirate patch and going from bird baths to a real shower. I rejoiced in the ability to wash my hair for the first time, any gap between the pain and discomfort, and the sanctuary of a sweet dream. Joy leapt with each day of no treatment. It resided in the miracle of my breath and my body's amazing capacity to heal. Joy filled me when I embraced the gift of every precious day.

The journey of our lives will propel us on many ups and downs. Without an inner connection to joy, we will be tossed around the sea of life like a piece of driftwood. We will feel the victim of every life circumstance. We have the choice of always relating to everyone with a sense of joy that comes from our inner being, despite how we physically feel or what challenge awaits us.

Joy comes from trusting that all will be good in the 360° picture of our lives, and every situation is a chance to practice that faith. Joy is born from love, kindness, and gratitude. There is joy even within our darkest hour, since joy is taking delight in simply being alive.

Joy is not happiness. Happiness is a roller-coaster ride. Joy is the deep kernel of truth and a blessing, seemingly hidden within each situation.

The choice is ours. Choose joy.

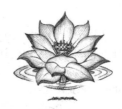

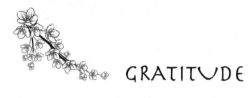

# GRATITUDE

"Life is effort."
So says the body.
"Life is blessing."
So says the soul.
-Sri Chinmoy

Gratitude unlocks the fullness of life. It turns what we have into enough,
and more. It turns denial into acceptance, chaos to order, confusion to clarity.
It can turn a meal into a feast, a house into a home, a stranger into a friend.
-Melody Beattie

For the last year and a half, every day has felt like Thanksgiving. Not the kind with cornucopias, carved turkeys, cranberries, and falling asleep from overeating, but the kind that resonates deep in my heart with immense gratitude for the blessings given, loving gifts received, and for the miracle of life itself.

A fourteen hour surgery, a missing ear, facial and spinal accessory nerves severed, muscles and nerves spliced, flaps of nodes removed, facial paralysis, limited movement, treatments, more surgery: The list goes on. One might wonder, how has this, then, been a time of great thanksgiving? How does anyone give thanks amid the assault of surgery, the crackling rays of radiation, the drip of chemotherapy, the unknowns of prognosis, the merry-go-round of side effects, and the realities of a "new normal"? How do we give thanks amid any of life's challenges?

We see what we look at. Do we stare at our insults and injuries, or our blessings and opportunities? Do we live asking "why me," or the truth of "why not me"? Do we focus on our pain and bitterness, or the awe and the wonder that surrounds us? Do we live in fear, or open up so we can experience all the love in our lives? The gifts are there, if we only look in their direction.

For the last year and a half, I saw great gifts of giving everywhere I looked and have felt great gratitude. I'm thankful for the giving, from things as seemingly small as a gentle touch on a weakened body, or the silence between the barks of the neighbor's dog as I lie in pain, to the immensity of a clear PET scan and the love of family and friends. I see endless prayers, positive thoughts, words of encouragement, acts of love, kindness, generosity, and the miracle of my healing.

It seems to me that the question and challenge for us all is: Can we be thankful for whatever life brings us? Can we not label good or bad, and then be open to see the gifts within our circumstances? In giving thanks, we can bow to each situation as our teacher.

Thanksgiving is just one day. Thanks and giving are each day. Words fall short when expressing deep gratitude. My Team Suzette family and friends continually keep me in their light, hold me in their hearts, embrace me with their prayers, surround me with their positive thoughts, shower me with their kindness, fill me up with their generosity, and saturate me with their love.

Let us all embrace, cherish, and give thanks for all our gifts, whatever our circumstances, whatever our path. Let our challenges remind us to move into a wider expanse of the heart. Let us connect more deeply with all of life, experience joy, embrace the moment, and appreciate the journey. Let us remain humbled by all the immense divine blessings in our lives and know that everything matters.

Although there are many small and big things that I continue to be incredibly thankful for, I am especially appreciative of the great gift of the Affordable Care Act. While many throw daggers and darts in his direction, I will forever have great gratitude to President Obama and the passing of this legislation. I would never have been able to get the insurance that has allowed me to be treated at the City of Hope with my preexisting condition. As a single, self-supporting woman, the tax credits granted me reasonable premiums for my income. The cost of fourteen hours of surgery at the hands of gifted surgeons, a long hospital stay, countless appointments, procedures, biopsies, scans, radiation, chemotherapy, appointments, additional surgeries, and physical therapy afterward would have been galaxies away from my financial reach. Everyone at City of Hope that reads my file says what an over-the-top surgery was performed in those fourteen hours, and how those three surgeons went to bat for me 110 percent that day. Thank you President Obama, and thanks to all of those individuals and groups that worked so hard for decades to make the Affordable Care Act a reality and so become a part of saving my life.

Let us always ask ourselves: What can I be grateful for at this present moment in time? If we rest in stillness and openness, we will see many gifts before us. Gratitude was spread out like an inviting welcome mat throughout my journey. I gave thanks for the mechanics of the hospital bed positioning my body, the eye I could see out of, a soft boiled egg sliding down a raw throat, and the bolting of the radiation mask with a touch more space to breathe. I was grateful for a soft breeze against my body and every gift of sleep. Appreciation filled me during the parts on the roads that were not bumpy on the way to City of Hope. I rested in gratitude revisiting and now reading cards that were once read to me. I gave thanks whenever I didn't have to think, was surrounded by silence, and when neighbors turned off their late night rap music. My heart was full of gratitude for all the money raised to help buoy me during my recovery. I said thank you when the swelling on my face softened into a more familiar Suzette in the mirror. Appreciation filled me when I could lift a saucepan on my own and with my first cut into my art materials after the removal of the sling. I was deeply thankful for the visits from my nieces and nephews and for every person who chauffeured me to the hospital. Each morning I gave thanks to my healing backyard sanctuary of plants, flowers, and wildlife. I rested in eternal thanks for a deeply loving village of family and friends and amazing grace. One thought of gratitude creates a hundred more.

If we want more happiness, joy, and energy, we must rest in gratitude. Why do we so often rest in complaint and bitterness? Gratitude is the fullness of heart that allows our limitations and fears to lessen, disappear, and then expand into love. When we're appreciating something, we get out of our own way to connect with a deeper source. Gratitude brings our attention to the beauty in whatever is happening right now. This is the place of miracles. The deeper our gratitude, the more our life flows in harmony with the creative power of the universe. The wider we open, the deeper we fall into the healing arms of love. Finding gratitude lightens our load and makes the journey one of our eternal heart, not our ever-changing body.

When we are hooked to a chemotherapy bag, or strapped into the radiation tunnel, how can we be grateful? We can give great thanks for the smile and compassion of the nurse, the research that went into developing the hoped-for cure, the areas of health and strength within our body, a few hours of quiet, meditative silence, and our blessed insurance that makes our recovery financially possible.

In finding gratitude, we bow to every circumstance as our teacher. We offer thanks to every experience as part of the merry-go-round ride of our life. Eventually we not only have appreciation for our families, friends, our body, our doctors and their staff, and each person that offered words of encouragement or gifts of generosity, but also for the illness or life situation itself, for its insights and lessons.

If I was to really say yes and rest in immense gratitude, then I knew I had to find it also within the gifts of the "illness" itself. In this spirit, and straight from my heart, I expressed appreciation to the diagnosis. This was written not with the intent to write great poetry, but to express deep thanks to the cancer for its blessings.

## A THANK YOU NOTE TO MY DIAGNOSIS

Thank you...
For stripping me to the core,
sinking me even deeper
into the pure ocean of truth.

For the months of meditative silence
where lines between form and spirit dissolved
to feel the connection between everything and everyone.

For seeing the divine in the face of all nature
The flight of the birds, the whimsy of the squirrels
and the tiniest ant making its way across the patio.
For narrowing my aperture
and slowing life to a freeze frame
so I could sense the bud bursting into bloom.

Feel the wind before it blows.
Hear the silence and so the voice of God.

Thank you for all the tender moments...
A held hand and each "I love you."
A nephew saying, "I would take this pain from you if I could."
For my sisters' words and action to "have my back."
For every time my finger rested on the belt loop of loved ones,
guiding me in my weakness and impaired vision.
For each and every act of kindness and generosity.

Thank you for
allowing me to know pain
so I can be ever more compassionate
to those who carry their own.

Thank you...
For all the small joys over these months
that felt like fireworks exploding
in the dark of my night sky.

Thank you...
For the doctors who worked so diligently, expertly,
and compassionately to remove you
For every prayer
For every positive thought
For the miracle that is.

For the tidal wave of love that crashed on my shore
The knowing that love
is truly the healing force
For opening my heart even wider
to experience that giving and receiving love
is the essence of our lives.

Thank you...
For the knowledge that no matter what the seeming
darkness, the light is there.
That to follow even the hint of its memory
can lead to brilliance and illumination.

Thank you...
For the bone and marrow experience
that everything changes.

For the reminder to breathe even deeper
into the gift of each day.

For the example of the body's amazing ability to heal
and that you can totally leave
with no trace of footsteps left behind.

Thank you...
For all that was done for me without my asking
but rising from loving thoughtfulness.

For the experience of a deeply loving family
who became my eyes, my hands, and my engine.
For Team Suzette,
who carried me on the wings of their love.

Thank you...
For the reminder each time I look in the mirror
and see my paralyzed, grafted face
that I am not the garment of my body
but an eternal soul connected to all souls.

For my surrender to the bigger picture,
letting go of the attachment
to everything and anything, even my life,
for what is the highest possible divine good and will.

Thank you for leaving...
for bowing out of this dance we have been on
so I can now dance with joy, wild abandon, and deeper truths
in an ever closer embrace with life.

For allowing the neck of the hourglass
to widen into infinity and expand into nothing but blue skies.
Thank you for leaving
and giving me my life
where I will remain in endless gratitude

for all that I have received,
return the love that has been given to me, and
continue to enjoy this vast playground and schoolhouse.

Thank you for leaving.
For recognizing that the lessons have been learned
and are now ready to be even more deeply lived.
For giving me the opportunity to share my experience,
paint the blank canvas of each day,
and move from inner depths to the broad horizon.

Finally,
Thank you for staying away forever,
for living on the far side of the moon,
and so being a part of the continuous miracle of my healing.
And for all the precious totally and completely healthy
present moments that now unfold before me
to create the amazing tapestry of my life.

With gratitude comes joy and with joy comes gratitude. Celebrate your life. Celebrate right here, right now, and rest in thanks with whatever this moment brings to you. Appreciate all the beauty, grace, miracles, love, and light that is in front of you. They are always there. We need only open our eyes and our hearts. Let our joy and gratitude continue to open us to deeper healing.

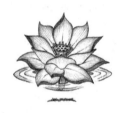

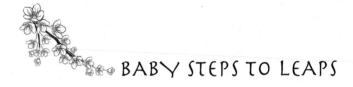

# BABY STEPS TO LEAPS

*It is better to take small steps in the right direction
than to make a great leap forward only to stumble backwards.*
*-Proverb*

Baby steps often feel like no progress—so small that they are some-times unnoticeable. However, baby steps create great leaps, which create the milestones of our journey. My leaps of progress along the way have been made possible by trusting each baby step, some notice-able to others and some noticeable only to me. All big triumphs, no matter how small. My head is able to make a slight turn to the right. I am blessed with the gift of a nap. I scramble an egg with one hand. Every so often, our baby steps become a leap that catches us unaware and reminds us of how far we have traveled on our journey. We must always keep our gaze on our triumphs, however small. Do not take the time to look backward. We must focus on what we can do by finding joy in each baby step, which takes us slowly but surely in the direction of our dreams and visions fulfilled.

All of my baby steps slowly become great leaps. After my surgery I walk down the hospital's corridor, to tenuously walking back and forth across my patio. I then maneuver myself along the walkway outside my house, to triumphantly venturing four doors down. I grad-ually walk the entire street with guidance and sporadic rests, to small nature hikes on flat trails with friends.

My practice of tai chi during recovery was simplified into just the breath and meditative stillness. Gradually, I am able to use my left hand to do very small movements using the inhale and exhale. With the sling finally off and the beginnings of physical therapy, my great triumph is to lift my right arm from my side to navel level. Slowly, with focus, discipline, and determination, I am able to execute the tai chi "integration breath" with my arms rising to heart level.

I hold a pencil tenuously in my left hand and make a spirited effort to create legible scribbles with this non-dominant side. With great focus and concentration, my left hand begins to print out short, one-word lists. One day, I write an entire somewhat legible note with my efforts as a gallant lefty. My sling is finally off, so I slowly write with my right hand again, pausing for ice compresses as the movement triggers ever-changing sensations in my neck and shoulder. I begin to peck on the computer keyboard with one hand through one blurry eye, and then, for short intervals, with both hands. Slowly but carefully, I work up to sending out the Team Suzette updates on my own.

Others clean for me, cut my vegetables, and cook my food. It is then a triumph to begin to steam broccoli with the help of their slicing and dicing. I gradually begin to cut soft foods on my own, and once again I am able to slice through my beloved avocados with my right hand.

I suck pureed food through a straw into the tiny hole that is my mouth's opening. With time, I am able to rest a small amount of blended food on a tiny spoon that makes its way carefully into my mouth. Eventually, I cut soft food into tiny pieces and use a fork or chopsticks to bring it up to my small opening. With more time and practice, I can fit bigger amounts into my mouth with less and less ending up on my lap. The day comes when I sit across from my family at a local restaurant and eat slowly, carefully, with adaptations, and without much embarrassment to anyone.

A toothbrush will not enter my mouth. Eventually a child's Minnie Mouse brush is able to enter sideways to reach a few teeth. With physical therapy, the opening widens and I am able to brush more and then more teeth with the small toothbrush.

Tidal waves of nausea are triggered by a slight movement or a few brief words. I eat a gulp of almond butter, a sip of soup, a soft boiled egg, or sometimes not at all. Then two gulps, two sips, or even two eggs. I begin to look at an avocado as appealing and finally, little bites are occasionally sliding down my throat. A full meal returns, then another. With baby steps, I begin eating breakfast, lunch, and dinner with avocados adorning each meal.

For six months I create no art, barring a few sketches with a willing but shaky left hand and one eye. I don't know if I will ever be able to create my art again. The sling comes off and, with scissors in hand, I slowly cut through my mixed media materials, rest, ice, and cut again. Baby steps. A small panel called *Courage* representing a theme from my healing journey, slowly and with adaptations, comes to life in my mixed media medium. Tenuously creating one image at a time, months later there are twenty-seven panels that become the 4.5′ × 5.5′ artwork entitled *The Journey is Everything*. It is purchased by my sister and her husband, Richard and Jeannine Lambert, as donors who believed that it needed to have a public showcase to inspire others throughout their healing. It now resides at the Long Beach Miller Children's & Women's Hospital in the Jonathan Jacques Children's Cancer Unit.

With faith, perseverance, and discipline, baby steps become visions fulfilled. We embrace each moment-to-moment baby step with patience and triumph, while also holding the vision of our own healing horizon. Then comes the day when we are standing in the reality of our cherished destination.

Several decades ago, I was drawn to the travel section at the San Diego Public Library. I was working full-time as the director of a center for teenagers, but wanderlust had begun to catch me unaware. Sitting on the floor of the library, I pulled out a book entitled *Guide to Unusual Vacations*. Flipping through its pages, they seemed to stop on their own at a picture of a hot air balloon going over the Swiss Alps. Craggy majestic peaks were covered deep in snow with hot air balloons billowing into take-off, and others mere dots fading into the morning sky. I wanted to be there. I saw myself there. Six months later, I began my solo adventure to wherever my heart and wallet would take me. Four months into my travels, I stood knee-deep in snow in the Swiss Alps as hot air balloons rested on the ground like colorfully animated cartoons. The picture in the book and in my mind had become the reality of my life at that moment. Since then, I have cherished those moments of standing in a dream fulfilled. As we travel the path to recovery, we receive precious gifts when our baby steps and dreams become our visions fulfilled. Our patience and moment-to-moment healing then catches us unaware. We find that we are indeed living in real time what was once an image in our mind.

Lying in bed with little ability to move, dancing with pain, confined and challenged with each breath, my vision was to be strong enough by year's end to spend some days and nights at the ocean's edge. I longed for the smell of the surf to flood every cell, the sound of the waves to lull me to sleep at night, to walk leisurely on the sand, and to silently watch the sun surrender itself to the horizon. Six months later, to celebrate our mutual birthdays, my sister and her wife took me on a road trip to Cambria to stay in a beautiful hotel with a balcony that overlooked jutting cliffs and a sparkling ocean. We spent three days watching the world pass by in all its wonder. There was a stillness that created timelessness, natural beauty that silenced words, and sea lions, deer, and otters who played with abandon in their natural turf. Vision fulfilled.

During the long, dark, and winding tunnel of treatment, another sister told me about the Walk to Cure Epilepsy, several months away. She has heroically been dealing with the challenges of epilepsy since childhood. Finally having surgery in her forties after no other medication had truly worked, she is now faced with the daily challenges of operating without a temporal lobe.

My vision was to walk beside her and be a part of "Team Jeannine." Four months later, I joined her and other family members to walk (stroll, rest, and stroll again) by her side to support her and the cure for epilepsy. A vision fulfilled!

One month after the end of my treatment, my sensei said he would be honored if I would perform a demonstration and write an essay for my fourth degree black sash in tai chi. My gears jammed. "What?" I had a patch over one eye, right arm was just out of the sling, and my movement was compromised along with the challenges of stamina and balance. I'd been out of the dojo for six months. Then I took a breath. "Why not?" The truth was that I had been in a marathon training for yondan, a fourth degree black sash, throughout my healing journey. My recovery was steeped in all the tai chi principles of deeply connecting with the breath, moment-to-moment living, continuing patience, unending meditative practice, moving slowly, staying open, and experiencing the power of immense love. Fourth degree black sash level is about the deeper understanding of tai chi, which holds the forms and our lives together. The test, to me, would represent the miracle of my being alive and my continual recovery at that moment in time. I had a vision of energy flowing through me with my heart wide open as I made my presentation to the dojo.

After six weeks of hard physical therapy to execute some of the moves (with adaptations due to my severed spinal accessory nerve), and surrounded by the loving chi of my sensei and all the students, I shared an essay on the meaning of Yondan to me and a medley of forms, ending with Jimmy Cliff singing: "You can get it if you really want but you must try, try and try, try and try, you'll succeed at last." Truly a vision fulfilled.

After my surgery, I was mostly horizontal, drains in place, restricted in movement, limited in energy, and soon to begin radiation and chemotherapy. Our dojo's thirty-third annual retreat, which I have attended every year since I started my training almost twenty years ago, seemed so far away. Yet it was brought so close to my heart. Sensei Frank dedicated the retreat to my recovery and donated the proceeds to help with all things financial. A group of students brought Mt. Baldy to me through pine cones, rocks, and driftwood. Above all, a rock from the mountain that read "Mt. Baldy 2014" was given to me. With it was an incredibly moving video. I watched, in tears, as this rock was held in everyone's hands and infused with all their love, prayers, healing chi, and positive thoughts. I would often hold it in my palms after my chemotherapy infusions to also be infused with all its love. My vision was to be on the mountain at the next retreat, return the rock and have my sensei write "Mt. Baldy 2015" on it, breathe the healing air, surround myself with stillness, and thank everyone for their love and being a part of the miracle of my healing.

I returned to Mt. Baldy the following year. I embraced the retreat in gentle training with the senseis, walking in unison with the monks at the light of dawn, cherishing the opportunity to be heart-to-heart and face-to-face with everyone, and expressing my deep love and gratitude for all that was given to me. A vision fulfilled.

I will deliver that rock back to the mountain for many years to come. I will have Sensei Frank write each unfolding year on it with ink until it is covered in black and I'm forced to hand him a white pen.

No matter where we are in our journey—peak or valley—we must keep our vision toward our dreams. When we move in alignment with our own light, our highest physical, emotional, and spiritual energy, and our divine purpose, the creative infinite energy of the universe moves with us.

Great leaps and milestones are made from baby steps. We must not rush our healing. We need to surrender to the moment and rest in all we can do each inch of the way. Time takes on another meaning in the face of recovery. Healing is not measured with a linear or predictable trajectory. We must respect the body's need to go deeply within to heal, trusting that each baby step is building up to a great bound. If we can indeed embrace the now, then we aren't in a rush to get anywhere. Our society is on fast-forward, but we can move with divine time. If we can let go of fear, we can relax and accept that we are just where we need to be at each moment.

We don't give in to any voice to rush our healing. We treasure the baby steps as they keep us from being overwhelmed, knocked off balance, or triggered by a setback. Sometimes we rest just where we are; other times, we take a baby step forward. Everything takes courage, risk, and a trust in the unknown.

We are a work in progress. During our recovery, perhaps the only constant we feel is change, even hour to hour. We must take baby steps as little bits of our energy are slowly building and exploring different places in our body to heal. Our accelerators have been pushed into overdrive for months with all the myriad treatments. Baby steps are our body's testimony to us that it is slowly building its own ground, stamina, and reserves. Let go of the calendar. All healing takes place in the lap of timelessness.

Our progress can suddenly catch us unaware. Something that took too much energy before can now be done with more ease. The food slowly looks a bit more appealing on our plate. Side effects soften and then fade or even disappear. We learn to take our baby steps in peace and not frustration. We don't look backward to what was, but give great thanks to what is. We change our tune from "I used to be able to" to "I can do this." We adjust to a new reality that is actually, in fact, what any one of us are doing for each unfolding moment of our lives.

Celebrate the baby steps. Allow them to become leaps. We climb the highest mountain peak one step at a time. Leaps become the visions fulfilled. Visions fulfilled become the beautiful, broad brush strokes of our healing, as well as an ongoing testimony to the strength of our mind, body, and spirit.

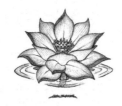

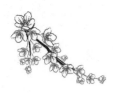

# EXPECT A MIRACLE

Accept your diagnosis, but not your prognosis.
-Deepak Chopra

Miracles are not contrary to nature,
but only contrary to what we know about nature.
-St. Augustine

The invariable mark of wisdom is to see the
miraculous in the common.
-Ralph Waldo Emerson

There are only two ways to live your life. One is as though
nothing is a miracle. The other is as if everything is.
-Albert Einstein

I have a huge stack of medical reports from before my surgery and needed to sort through them to find some needed documentation. I happened to glance at a report by the oculo-facial surgeon when she had first examined my eye for a potential skin graft. She was listing the history of my surgery and ensuing treatment. Then the next line read: "And her PET scan is now miraculously clear." The word *miracle* jumped off the paper and did a high dive into the depths of my heart. How often does a doctor use the word miracle? Much less include it in her report to other doctors?

That word wouldn't be on the medical report without the wings of Team Suzette. Prayers, love, faith, encouragement, positive thoughts, compassion, the expertise of my doctors, treatments, and the grace of the divine brought forth the miraculous. It is not for us to understand where miracles come from. It is only for us to believe in them.

What are miracles? As a child growing up in the Catholic Church, miracles were always about huge acts of wonder, such as the healing at Lourdes, the children of Fatima seeing the Virgin Mary, Jesus walking on water, and his resurrection from the dead. We look for miracles when our life circumstances screech to a halt. We pray for a miracle when a loved one is seriously ill or faces a life-threatening challenge. We ask for them, but we often do not believe they truly exist or doubt we are deserving. However, miracles are not few and far between. They are not given out in small doses every century or two. They are not for someone else instead of us. They are not confined to the person in a wheelchair who gets up to walk, or the mute person who suddenly starts to speak. We put miracles in a box. However, the miraculous cannot fit into any box. If we limit ourselves to the fears about our future, there is no room for miracles. Instead, if our minds and hearts remain open in awe and wonder, then we will see and experience them every day. If we set aside our ego's need to control and understand, and are totally open to whatever comes our way through infinite grace, then miracles large and small will arrive at the open door to our heart. When we embrace an experience and expect wondrous things, we won't be disappointed.

Thich Nhat Hahn, the great Buddhist monk, said, "The true miracle is not to walk either on water or in thin air, but to walk on earth. Every day we are engaged in a miracle which we don't even recognize. A blue sky, white clouds, green leaves, the black curious eyes of a child, our own two eyes. All is a miracle." Standing on the mat in my dojo for the first time after my surgery and treatment, expressing my love and gratitude, was a miracle. Attending my own fundraiser was a miracle. Being at the Harmony Art Fair and the Hillcrest Festival of the Arts surrounded by my artwork and all those who came to visit was indeed a miracle. A clear PET scan was a miracle. Small miracles make up the big miracle of how far we have come in our healing. Some miracles happen instantly, while others unfold like a bud, slowly making its way to blossom. Miracles are the gifts we are given to provide a peephole beyond our very confined box we call reality. How often do we suffocate the awesome with fears, useless predictions, and old ways of thinking? Love is at the heart of every miracle. The beauty of love is that it is without limitation. Neither illness, life circumstance, nor money can keep us from opening our hearts. Without limitations, love flows and miracles happen.

As a Catholic student in a public elementary school, we took part in a "religious release" program once a week. Every Tuesday afternoon, a woman would escort us from our classroom to her home a block away. We were to spend an hour receiving a "booster shot" of our Catholicism to "vaccinate" us from being in the perhaps contagious and irreligious environment of a public school. One afternoon, we all sat on a picnic bench in her backyard. Our teacher slowly placed an acorn, a seed, and a picture of a newborn on the table. She asked us if we had ever experienced a miracle. We all assured her we had only read about them in books. She pointed to all the items on the table and told us that we were staring face to face with the miraculous. The tiny acorn became the huge oak tree towering over us. The small seeds transformed into the watermelon she had cut and sliced for our snack. The picture of the tiny newborn was her, and now she was standing before us as a grown woman. "We are surrounded by miracles every-day. You are a miracle. God's miracles are within everything in the universe." For each chapter of my life, I experience her words at deeper and deeper levels. I now indeed feel like a miracle.

Some people long each day for the grand fireworks of miracles to explode before them. Some look for a miracle only when circumstances are life-threatening. Many wish their lives away waiting for that great, miraculous future moment. Truly, every day is a miracle.

We need only to put on a lens of openness, courage, and vulnerability so we are fully awake to the miracles within and throughout. In the hubbub of our lives, everything can become a blur. Within the fears and anxieties of our diagnosis and treatment, we often close down. Distracted by the ever-revolving door of thoughts in our mind, we lose sight of the miraculous, never getting the miracle of each precious moment back. When we rest in stillness and silence, we begin to see miracles right in front of us. It is a miracle to be alive. It is a miracle to be spinning on this planet at this moment in time. It is a miracle that in our fragility we are also so strong. The healing on the other side of suffering and illness is a miracle. It is a miracle that the sun rises and sets and is held in vast, precious space by the invisible hands of the infinite. The Earth spins on its axis, bringing us from dawn to dusk and from expansive light to the depths of darkness. The seasons have unfolded for centuries with perfect rhythm and elegant effortlessness. Moments of great kindness miraculously touch us. A smile or the unexpected, small gift of a stranger can feel miraculous in its timing. Each of the billions of people on this planet are their own individual blueprint, as special and unique as each flower, tree, animal, and bird. Our birth from a sperm and an egg to life is miraculous. Instruments made of random wood, wire, and copper can be put together to strum, blow, or tap to move us to an avalanche of emotional depth. Our body is a miracle: each cell, each breath, and each beat of the heart. The healing power of love and deep friendship is miraculous. How can anyone look at the majesty of the world and see its wonder, awe, immense beauty, overwhelming creativity, endless palettes of color, and divine timing and not be shaken by the miraculous?

My mother saw the miraculous in everything. She called all the amazing grace and unexpected gifts in her life her "MMs" (Major Miracles). When smaller acts of wonder and love entered her life, they were her "mms" (minor miracles). When she took my sister and I on a trip to our homeland in Ireland, six months before her spirit soared, she saw miracles everywhere. They were so abundant that we began to make lists dividing them into major and minor miracles. There was the divine timing of being in her beloved priest's childhood church in Ireland on the exact Sunday morning he was on vacation there giving the mass. Our seemingly futile search for our great-grandmother's gravestone in a cemetery was about to end when a woman walking her dog reached out to visit with us, sharing that she passed the tombstone every day. Belief and miracles go hand in hand. If we are not open to them, they cannot flow into our lives. Her belief and gratitude for the miracles in her life seemed to bring them to her. My mother would indeed deem my healing as a front-runner in her list of Major Miracles.

My kitty Tattoo never ceased to amaze me with her more than nine lives. She taught me to never limit yourself or anyone else by fearing a future prognosis. Time after time, the vet gave predictions on her life that soon became meaningless. Perhaps Tattoo's miracles, and a cat's nine lives, come from not suffocating the possible with thoughts of the impossible. Cats are the masters of being in the moment, relaxed, and at peace. Miracles can then flow through them because they are open to the miraculous, not confined by the possible, harrowing scenarios and predictions about their future.

Expect an MM—a MAJOR MIRACLE!

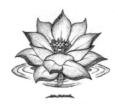

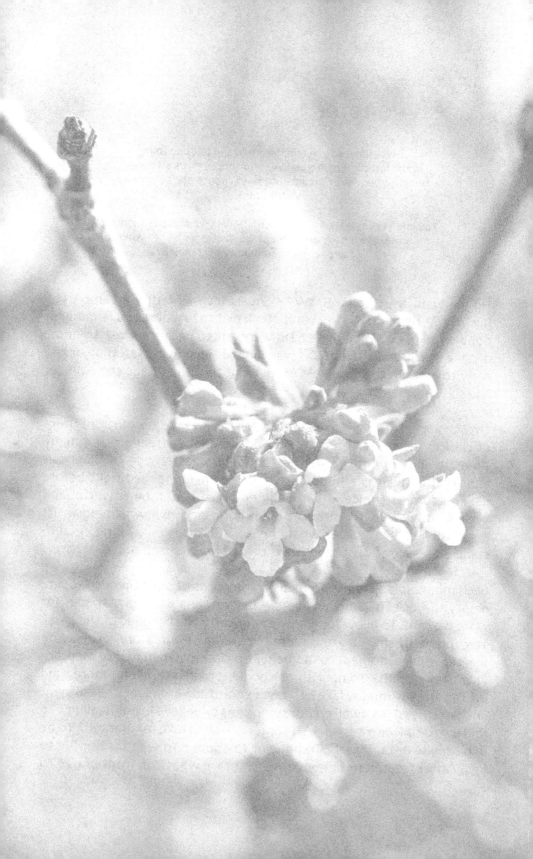

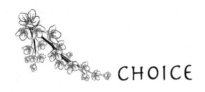

# CHOICE

Everything can be taken from a man but one thing:
the last of human freedoms—to choose one's attitude
in any given set of circumstances, to choose one's own way.
-Victor Frankl

You and I are essentially infinite choice-makers. In every moment
of our existence, we are in that field of all possibilities where
we have access to an infinity of choices.
Deepak Chopra

Do we want a VW or a BMW? Convertible or hardtop? Lemon yellow or mystic blue? Do we want steak or fish? Apple pie à la mode or double fudge chocolate cake? Do we want to vacation close to home or take a cruise to Alaska? Do we want to sleep in on Saturday or rise early to work in the garden? Do we want to retire at age sixty-two or age sixty-six?

Often we feel that these kinds of questions make up our repertoire of choices in life. However, we have tremendous freedom and many times it goes unnoticed during the roller-coaster ride of diagnosis and treatment. It is a huge gift that remains unopened right before us. Freedom of choice, if we really embrace it, can be powerful and life-changing, but it can also be daunting and overwhelming in its responsibility. No matter what the horrific or awe-inspiring circumstances are, we always have the choice of how to respond.

Each moment is a choice. To focus on the locus of our pain or the open, empty spaces? To complain about what we can't do or give thanks for what we can? To allow for a new day or carry the baggage of the past? To continually sink into and share the drama of our "story" or recreate our experience moment to moment? To close down in fear or embrace in trust and faith? To nourish our bodies or keep throwing more mud into an already muddy lake? To rest in gratitude or fall into resentment and bitterness? To dwell on our symptoms or believe in our healing? To find joy or sink into despair? To appreciate or to take for granted? To be in our mind or our heart? To hope or to doubt? To wait for our life to begin after treatment or honor and embrace what is in front of us? To learn to find the light within our circumstance or withdraw into the darkness? To be a victim or a warrior?

Suffering ceases to be suffering at the moment it finds meaning. We have choices each day throughout our journey of healing and our lives. Moment to moment, we decide how we are to respond to the challenges life places before us. Moment to moment, we create our thoughts and our actions. Moment to moment, we can choose to bring meaning to our experience.

It may seem as if we are left without a choice during our diagnosis and our recovery. We exclaim: I didn't choose this! And then we ask: What choice do I have? A port or no port? The needle in my wrist, or inside the crook of my elbow? Chemotherapy, radiation, or both? Shall I maneuver the hospital bed to the left or the right? Should my next appointment be on a Monday or Wednesday? How long should I lie down each day in fatigue? However, when it feels like we have lost all control in the midst of diagnosis and treatment, that is also when our power of choice gains its greatest strength and momentum. Within the supposed constraints of recovery also blooms much freedom. Since stress is not what happens to us, but how we respond to what happens to us, we are continually given the great freedom of how we will react to each unfolding moment. Our healing journey then becomes a master class of on-the-spot challenges, pop quizzes, and deep lessons. We are continually asked to respond to our circumstances, either with frustration and bitterness, or with openness and a gentle spirit of appreciation for each person in our village, as well as each circumstance along our healing path.

Sometimes our choices can feel like the difference between life and death. Sometimes they are the difference between life and death. Do we continue with treatment or stop? Do we have surgery or not? My decision not to have the remaining suspicious nodes removed after my treatment was a big choice. However, the endless and seemingly small choices before us actually hold the most power. What do we choose to say to ourselves in the dark of the night and when we open our eyes to a new day? Do we smile and give thanks to the volunteer who escorts us to the elevator, the receptionist who checks us in, the nurse who draws our blood, and the doctor who reveals our test results? Do we choose to breathe deeply into the present moment, or continually choose to let our minds fast-forward into the fear of an unknown future? Do we wait in the medical office with patience and understanding for our name to be called or do we fall into frustration and bitterness? Do we choose to smile or look away from those who pass us by in the hallway, dragging their IV stands behind them? Do we rest in "why me" or "why not me"? Each choice is ours and ours alone.

Viktor Frankl's wife, father, mother, and brother died in the concentration camps of Nazi Germany. Frankl himself was in constant threat of being sent to the gas ovens as he endured extreme hunger, cold, and brutality. He lost all his physical belongings on his first day in the camp, including a scientific manuscript he considered his life's work.

Within the suffering of the concentration camp, Frankl discovered the power of choice. Understandably, Frankl could have very easily believed his life was meaningless. Yet having been thrust into the depths of suffering, as the phoenix rising from ashes, he became an optimist. He was able to soar in the most terrible of circumstances by embracing the fact that he still had the freedom to choose how he would respond to his life, creating meaning from his challenging reality. He still had the power of choice.

Frankl was kept afloat by thoughts and visions that allowed him to connect with joy and purpose. Mental reminders of his wife lightened the suffocating darkness. Visions of sharing his experiences in imprisonment and life after liberation, as well as reconstructing his manuscript, were slivers of hope that shattered the darkness. Ultimately, even though he was in the most dire of circumstances, he could choose how he was going to respond, which gave him his freedom.

In each moment, we are deciding our future. Each moment is our point of power. In every moment, we determine the melody of our lives. We may not get the notes we want, but we can piece them together in our own melody and sing with inspiration or desperation. We can't control traffic on the way to the hospital, our test results, and the mood of the doctor or nurse, but we can control our response to every situation.

With our freedom of choice also comes great responsibility and letting go of blame. This is no easy task, as complaint, resentment, and fear have sometimes become our strange allies. If the choice in how we respond to everything is truly ours, then a life ridden with bitterness, fear, and misery is also due to our own choosing. We have to be willing warriors and give up our armor of blame in exchange for the freedom of wielding responsibility over our lives.

Wherever we place our attention determines what we see. That is the power of choice. Whatever we choose to both look at and say yes to answers us in agreement. We become one with the object of our choice. If we choose joy, we are one with truth, strength, and love. If we choose to keep our attention on our own small stories, we are isolated instead of connected to the true power of our source. Consequently, we suffer. The more we make choices for our greatest good, the better we feel. This continues until the balance in our lives begins to tip in favor of being at peace in the ever-present moment, rather than suffering in fear and separation. Our choices create our freedom or imprisonment. Ultimately, we have only one choice: Do we move from love or from fear?

If we choose to, we live in the truth that every thought and every action matters in the script of our lives. Then each moment we wield our power of choice with freedom and in gratitude. We choose to give all our moments in time meaning and hope, in illness or good health.

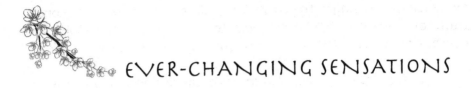

# EVER-CHANGING SENSATIONS

*Find a place inside where there is joy,*
*and the joy will burn out the pain.*
-Joseph Campbell

For almost every appointment since before my surgery, I have been asked to give a number between one and ten to reflect my pain level. This has been a continuing challenge for me. I like to think of "pain" as "ever-changing sensations." I don't like to give it an identity, numerical power, or a solid presence. Pain can be a demanding and strange bedfellow. It can be the first to greet me into the new day. In the middle of the night, it can come to wake me from my much-needed sleep as if it were afraid of the dark and in need of company. As I move through the day, it longs for me to put on the brakes and skid my activity to a stop. It wants definition, solidity, acknowledgment, and permanence. It is a spoiled child demanding my attention exclaiming: "Me! Me! Me!"

Like the rippling in a lake from one single stone toss, pain often has its secondary repercussions. There is the experience of the pain, but more importantly, there is often a conversation that takes place within us about the pain. This is a negative and ruminative discourse that builds on its own momentum. Pain can sing out loudly about its suffering, demanding our attention so we find it difficult to focus on the surrounding areas of soothing openness. It is often the proverbial squeaky wheel that gets the oil. However, pain is the physical sensation we experience: Our suffering is the story we give to the pain. Pain may be inevitable, but our suffering is not. Letting go of the conversation around our discomfort can be a letting go of some of our pain. What is the dialogue we have with our pain in the quiet dark of the night? What do we whisper in its ear? Do our words sink us deeper into the abyss of its grip? Do we find ourselves handing over our power to its incessant screams? Do we give it a strong and solid identity? Do we make it an inevitability through imagined scenarios of its future? Do we allow our words to slip us into a downward spiral of anxiety? Do we hear ourselves say, "The pain is so horrible. I can't go on much longer like this." Often we just say the word "pain" and we feel the contraction and the unforgiving tightness.

Our emotional response to pain can cause more suffering than the pain itself. We have such a strong desire for the pain to leave forever, but our frustrations and attachment to its departure only add more tension and stress. Our wild mind clasps onto each sensation in our bodies, creates a fearful thought, and doesn't want to let it go. It seeks definition, labels, and solidity.

So how do we best deal with the lyrics of our pain? How do we continue to tolerate every one of its changing sensations? How do we not tighten and stand guard? How do we say "yes" to our pain and accept the tugging, twisting, pulling, and firing that wants to proclaim: "I am here and I am not going anywhere." It is so important to create a new dialogue that turns the "I can't stand this!" into a more positive message. If I sang out a repeating chorus of "Ah, the muscle and nerve pain in my right shoulder and neck is overwhelming," I would indeed feel overwhelmed. However, if my lyrics were "Ah, my left side is so free and empty and open," I could feel a sense of reprieve. If I said "This pain is killing me," my body would recoil and contract. But if my words changed to "all is healing" or "this too shall pass" my body would open and soften. If we can break the pattern of our circuitous thoughts around the pain, we can often break the seeming solidity of the pain itself. Ultimately, with practice and love, we can change the lyrics of the "ever-changing sensations" to actually become a "thank you" and a reminder of the miracle and grace of being alive.

If we can change the rutted pattern that the mind creates around the pain, we are left with a flow of ever-changing sensations and the open vistas surrounding them. Focusing on the sensations in our body with a sense of mindfulness can offer us a reprieve. We can then feel what is happening moment to moment and notice that what we experience isn't a solitary mass. What are the sensations we feel? A tingling, aching, burning? A feeling of heat or cold? A tugging, twisting, and pulling? If we can look at the pain as an impartial observer without emotional attachment, then we lose the mind's tightened hold on our experience. When we don't give what is happening a solid name and just feel our body in the moment, our discomfort becomes several ripples of twists and aches instead of a tsunami. Calmly observing the pain in the moment destroys its future. We feel the ever-changing sensations and discover that these individual sensations are a much lighter load than the accumulated hard rock that we have labeled as our pain.

My practice has been to focus not on the scream of the pain, but on the areas of polite whispers surrounding it, where the volume knob is turned downward. Certainly I have also been the bad parent to this spoiled, whining child and while overwhelmed and exasperated, yelled "shut up!" Of course, like a child, it responds to my contraction and resistance by increasing its tension and persistence. This makes the pain feel like a concrete and fixed point of no return.

If we can slowly pull back and observe the physical and emotional sensations, we find the space within the pain. We realize that pain isn't our entire experience. We begin to focus on the areas around the pain with no sensations. We sense the entire vista of our body, not just the fenced in area of discomfort. We unlock the gate, open the door, and let the tightly clasped fist of pain open and flow into the vast horizon. We remove the piercing, close-up, micro-lens of pain and change to a panorama that allows everything to soften, widen, and become more manageable. We allow our breath to find its way into the contraction. We offer our pain the loving space to surrender and let go. We compassionately merge with it as we long to merge with the infinite. We let the turbulence of pain be engulfed by a vast space of calm.

In the middle of night, with nerves shooting and muscles pulling, it often seemed like there was no space left in my body. I would then make my way through the sliding glass door into the backyard, look up at the expanse of the starlit sky, and free-fall into its infinity. I sought to put healing space around whatever was happening and let the "ever-changing sensations" float and expand into the infinite galaxies. I would attempt to focus not on "the pain," but instead visualize all the seemingly hard and relentless sensations turning into vapor. At times, I would imagine my partner, Chuck, whom I longed to be here for this journey, holding my hand as I rested in his safe arms. Other times I would feel sweet Tattoo's peaceful presence, the love of family and friends, and the grace of the divine comforting me. I would seek to use the power of my mind to soothe the cries of my body.

When the days seemed like an eternity of nerves firing, muscles twisting, and everything happening in such a tightened space that even a slight contraction caused all to scream, the breathing would be my salvation. I would find the breath, connect with it, follow it, and gently guide it into the area to soften the sensations, if only for a millisecond. Just the breath. Just right here. Just right now.

Intense physical discomfort can be one of the most difficult things to answer with a "yes." It can be electrifying, horrifying, terrifying, and seemingly never-ending. In pain, we can feel isolated and helpless. However, saying yes to our pain is not an invitation for it to stay. It does not mean that we like our pain. It does mean accepting that it is there and not pushing it away, so we don't create more physical tension and stress. We let go of the added contraction of the "no" so we can begin to lessen the discomfort, no matter how little or seemingly nonexistent. The "ever-changing sensations" are still there, but the "yes" invites an expansiveness to surround the pain. We open up and can deeply feel the stillness and silence that reveals "I have the space to encompass everything." When the ominous clouds of our pain engulf us, we must seek to connect with the expansive blue sky, which can hold everything. In doing so we make friends with the pain instead of resisting it and giving it more power. The "yes" is the open door to relax around the contraction. We may desire the sensations to leave forever; however, saying yes is our acknowledgment that it exists right here, right now. We then send our pain love instead of hate, calm instead of anxiety, acceptance instead of denial, and the healing energy of the present moment instead of an imagined, solid, never-changing future.

When we feel pain, does it become a trigger to remember a previous time when we could move easier and with wilder abandon? Does it create a dialogue of "poor me" or "this will never end"? Do we allow it to be a voice to remind us to be thankful for the gift of our lives? Do we use the pain to connect deeper with our spirit and rest in calm and great hope? As always, the choice is ours.

If I focus on my body, I want it to be a reminder of its great strength, healing, and perseverance. I may not be what was, but I continue to be amazed at what is. As my dad always said when asked how he was: "Compared to what?" If I cling to wanting what was, I will suffer. Accepting, adapting, and learning from "what is" becomes my freedom. I am gradually discovering and creating new steps and routines for the best dance with my body, with its new challenges, movements, "ever-changing sensations," and energy. I bow to my body in deep respect and awe for all that it has experienced and all the ways it has healed. I am so blessed to continue to have a life abundant with joy, deep love, and unfolding opportunities.

We must listen to our body and its vast wisdom. We must remember that it is our friend, even when we are in pain. Whatever our experience is of pain, we must ask it: "What have you to teach me?" We must remember that the most important questions on our journey are: "What can I learn?" and "How can I open my heart wider?"

Let each throb, bolt of lightning, burn, twist, and ache be a reminder of the gift of each day and the miracle of being alive. Let us change our lyrics to ones of gratitude. Let the sensations sing out: "You are here. You are blessed." Let the "pain" be yet another reminder of the skill of our medical team, the love and compassion of our family and friends, and the grace of the divine for granting us this precious day.

Let us continually seek to soften into the moment, let go, and breathe deeply into right here, right now. Let us not isolate ourselves into solitary confinement with our pain. Let us not create a melodramatic story of our distress. Let us not get pulled into the force of its seeming black hole. Yes it can indeed be excruciating. However we must open up and rise above again and again, if only for a moment. Listen to your favorite music. Seek out quiet and stillness. Focus on the breath. Savor the smell and beauty of a flower and let it permeate every cell. Inhale open space, and exhale stress and contraction. No matter how intense the moment, remember we have been given the gift of being here. Reach out to someone instead of contracting inward. Say a prayer. Help someone in need. Sit in nature. Laugh. Find joy. Give or send love. Connect with the light that surrounds us and is us. Take gentle care of your body and spirit with a bubble bath, a massage, and deep rest. Seek out the gentle healing touch of a loved one. Remember that everything changes. Know that we are healing with every positive choice we make. We must keep reminding ourselves that we are not the constriction of our pain but the expansiveness of our spirit. And always remember that "this too shall pass."

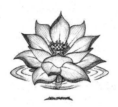

 TRUST

Consider the lilies of the field, how they grow. They neither toil nor
spin; yet I say unto you, even Solomon in all his glory was not
arrayed like one of these. And which of you by being anxious can
add a cubit unto the measure of his life?
-Matthew 6:28-27

Trying to fast-forward into the future jams my gears. I don't even
know how and what I will feel from hour to hour. I don't know the
new picture on the jigsaw puzzle of my life. All is definitely an improvisational melody and, time and time again, I try to practice the art of
living moment to moment. It is not always easy and sometimes I am
a dismal failure.

After the surgery I let everything go—driving, seeing out of both eyes,
how I looked, and what I could and couldn't do. I wasn't surrendering
and waving a white flag. It was not that I didn't care. I was letting go
and trusting that new things would replace whatever disappeared and
whatever returned would be a gift. So I let my life be a blank canvas. A
painting is magnificent, but a blank canvas is awaiting many things—
wonder, mystery, new beginnings, and new adventures.

It takes great courage to trust that our challenges will ultimately sink
us into a deeper growth and understanding. It takes great faith to trust
the journey to teach us what we need to learn. It takes much humility
to trust that what is before us is a gift, not a burden.

Trust means letting go of fear. Today is just the way it is supposed to
be. Letting go and trust are bedfellows. To trust the bigger picture
means letting go of the petty, the small, and even all that seems to
loom large and foreboding in front of us. It means extending the welcome mat to this moment in time.

When they discovered remaining suspicious nodes after the completion of my treatment, I had to choose between waiting a month to see if they progressed or immediately having them surgically removed. I decided to trust that my body could continue to heal them on its own. Living in trust is akin to the dot-by-dot connective pictures I used to love as a child. I could never predict beyond the current dot. I'd watch what I thought was the arm of a clown turn into the trunk of an elephant and finally into a tree filled with beautiful birds. The same is true with me. I have never known how the dots in my life will connect. I've always trusted the bigger picture, and I do so now. I trust it is one beautiful understanding that I can only partially see and comprehend in the moment. One thread does not reveal the entire tapestry. How many times in our lives has complete misfortune led to great beauty, transformation, and deep lessons? How often has the mud given us the lotus blossom? How frequent is it that what we have cursed became one of our most treasured blessings in the retrospective view of our lives? I try to capture more than an eyeful of the expansiveness around me, but my narrow sight sees only one tiny slice. My peripheral vision allows me to see to my left and to my right, but how much do I miss by not seeing the entire panorama? I am lulled at times by the security of my own small insights. I turn my head, sometimes a mere cock of the neck, and my world changes. I can never see the entire picture. The infinite sees in 360°, in 3D, and in color. I am but a camera with a fixed lens, only able to capture one frame at a time. Even if I turn slowly, little by little, piecing together all I see, I miss the understanding of the whole and often forget that I am one with the whole. Each fragment of time in our lives only makes sense in the bigger picture. As time passes, we have more of a widened view of our life. However, it only our mysterious free fall into eternity that pulls open the drapes to shine light on the intricate meaning of each moment. Gazing through my tiny peephole of humanity, I feel very humbled and grateful. I do not know where each step is taking me. I just need to trust the inspirational divine melody of my life.

As I went through treatment, I continued to trust that all the present-moment, crazy, and circuitous dots in my life would connect into a picture of myself as amazingly strong, healthy, and vibrant. I envisioned all unwelcome critters disappearing to the far side of the moon. As they say, you can't control the wind, but you can direct the sails. All of my sails throughout my journey were set toward Destination Cure.

One month later, after deciding to trust my body to heal versus the option of surgery, the unwelcome suspicious nodes had disappeared.

When we trust, we fall head first into the present moment and open our hearts to what is. We surrender to whatever falls in our path. We trust that the challenges we face will lead to new understanding, new opportunities, and new blessings. To live or to die is not necessarily the ultimate question or the important outcome. We trust that the divine purpose of our lives is unfolding for our greatest good, so we accept everything with grace and gratitude. We both accept the unknown bigger picture of our lives while bowing before this moment in time. We trust that our lives are a magnificent gift and not a punishment.

Any crack, however small, even if a little light shines through, is our path to follow. Survivors of any challenge are like the flowers that push through the hard cement to bloom between the pavement's tiniest opening. We must trust that we can fit through any crack and that the smallest opening leads to bright, healing illumination. The Chinese hànzì for crisis is two symbols, danger and opportunity. What is our opportunity within the crisis? As we get closer to the light, it gets brighter until it embraces us, and the opportunities within our challenges are revealed. We trust that we can always shine through any crack, or even the hint of one, and it will lead us to greater freedom.

During my journey, many wanted to know what I did not know, asking for timelines, commitments, and the when, what, and how of my unfolding life. Everything was asked with the best of intentions. Yet, there is no crystal ball as we walk through our own individual wilderness of healing. Whatever lies ahead always remains an unknown: a "don't know." Much wide open space is needed for recovery and also for new opportunities to unfold.

After our treatment is an important time to embrace emptiness, not rushing to put the jigsaw puzzle pieces of our lives back together in the same way. We need not default to what was, but trust the current evolution of our lives instead. This allows for deeper healing. We are different now. Each experience in life changes us. It can be refreshing to tear up the blueprint we created and held in a tight grasp for so long, so we can step with faith, awe, and trust into the unknown. If we trust the open and empty space, it can lead us to a different rhythm in our lives and to deeper lessons. There is no hurry. We don't really need to know where we are going. We really only just need to feel deeply where we are at right now. Like a great jazz musician, we can then move to an improvisational beat and, note by note, trust the path that unfolds before us.

In life, we are continually shedding layers and growing new skin. We must trust that each time we let go it will lead to deeper truth and understanding. So we let go in faith, knowing we will be guided if we remain aware enough to receive the signs. We trust each step without having to know the next. We trust this day in our lives, this day of treatment, this side effect, and the roller-coaster ride of each day, knowing that it will take us, breath by breath, deeper into ourselves.

We just need to keep showing up in our lives. There is no understudy. If we aren't there, no one is, and we are not alive. If we can breathe into each moment and thus be on the center stage of our life, we discover that everything matters and everything changes. We can choose, moment to moment, to be in the spotlight or hide backstage in the dark. If we trust, we do not choose fear and the familiar, but reach out to the world with great love, faith, and knowing that we are ultimately instruments of divine love.

During recovery when everything is changing, trust can seem elusive and not within our reach. There is so much that asks for our trust as we travel down our healing path. We must trust our doctors, trust the results, and trust our body. We must trust when we are rolled into surgery and when the needle pierces its way into our veins to provide a pathway for the steady drop of chemotherapy. When our appetite disappears, we must trust that it will return. When we awaken, and it takes all of our willpower to pull ourselves from beneath our covers, we must trust that our healing is still taking place. In the dark of the night, we must trust that the light is there. When the future looms forebodingly, we trust in the moment. When the results come in, we must trust the bigger picture. When we ride the waves of nausea, we trust that the tide will calm. When we feel like there is no tomorrow, we trust that we will regain our ground and heal deeply. When the medical bills mount, we trust that money will come. We trust and continue to let go, knowing we are not our bodies, but the love, spirit, and heart that is immune to change. We continue to trust this seeming misfortune, which teaches us precious lessons that become the greatest gifts of our lives.

We must continue to trust, let go, and remember that everything changes. Change is the garment we wear in our lives here and now. Change is a gift because it tears us open to go deeper and deeper into ourselves. Yet we are fickle friends. When all is good, we want nothing to change. When things are bad, we want everything to change. Change can toss us around in the sea of life like a piece of driftwood. However, in illness or in health, if we can trust and flow with it, we have an opportunity to connect more deeply to the unchangeable within us. Treatment and recovery brings us into a more microcosmic, face-to-face dance with life's ever-changing footsteps. When I lived in Boston, they used to say: "If you don't like the weather, wait ten minutes." This is often the motto of our journey. During our recovery, it can often feel like the only constant is change from day to day, hour to hour, and moment to moment. A "sludge" brain turns to clarity, overdrive slowly unwinds into a little grounded energy, and shifting nerve and muscle pain ease into moments of relief. As we move into the new "normal," we find that our treatments have left much debris and destruction in their wake. Between the morphine, antibiotics, anesthesia, chemotherapy, radiation, steroids, nausea medications, scans, and dyes, there is a toxic river flowing inside of us. For me, the triple whammy of the over the top surgery, followed by chemotherapy and radiation, followed by more surgery, made change seem moment to moment. However, no matter how I was feeling, I trusted that everything I was doing was healing, cleansing, balancing, and strengthening as I slowly began to exercise, drink more organic green veggies, take important supplements, get as much sleep as I could (all things considered), be out in nature, embrace what I love, and rest in stillness and meditation. It is important to go with the flow, trust in our body's amazing capacity to heal, and not give any symptom too much power. We heal inward so we can slowly reach outward to embrace each new day. We rest and trust in our body's ability to rebuild and renew as it creates the baby steps that transform into the leaps of our healing. When asked how I was doing during my healing journey, the answer was simply, "I'm in recovery to an amazing destination!"

Free-fall into trust. Trust that your body is healing. Trust yourself, your loving village, this moment, the unfolding of each day, and in the infinite. Surrender and let go.

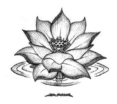

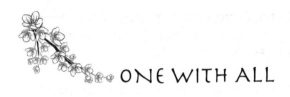# ONE WITH ALL

Our separation of each other is an optical illusion of consciousness.
-Albert Einstein

I look outward from my patio chair and see the flowers explode in color, fireworks in the daylight green of my backyard. Golden leaves of sunshine wave to me in the breeze and bushes hover over new blossoms like protective parents. Not unlike me, they went inward only to bloom again.

I see crisp clean lines that separate without shades of gray. This is a tree. There is the sky. Here is a potted plant. There are seemingly clear and defined lines between us. We live with boundaries of all kinds—each other, this country, that continent, and this galaxy. Boundaries crumble and fall when sitting for so long in healing, meditative stillness. We convince ourselves that we need them to give identity and meaning. This is my car, my house, my opinion, my family, and my belongings. We work so hard to separate, define, make special, compare, and contrast. We continually sharpen our individuality, like some glistening edge of a paring knife that oftentimes becomes too sharp for others to even draw near.

Where are my boundaries when I stand and say: "This is me. This is where I begin. Yes, you are there, but I am here." Quiet, solitude, and stillness tune us to a different frequency. I pause to look beyond the dotted lines and can feel the clutter of life fall away. Petty details fade, insignificant clingings drop, useless arguments leave, and small failures end. I see where everything melts into one. I see where love and gratitude expand into an endless circle. It is not a linear, separate world. Mystery, passion, creativity, and love live within sorrow and confusion. The forest is also the clearing, the argument and the resolution unite, the pulling away and the hug are one, joy and sorrow merge, and birth and death remain a revolving door to eternal life. Our constant chatter of individual voices wants to be heard, but in our silence, heart-to-hearts, and soul-to-souls, we are one. In our last moments, all boundaries disappear and everything and everyone blends into eternity.

My healing is everyone's healing. Everyone's joy is my joy. Our sorrows belong to each other. Every individual ripple we create changes the tide for all of us in this ocean of life. The tide of Team Suzette carries me in its warm, healing, and loving current. Deep gratitude resides in me for each individual ripple of kindness, generosity, love, prayer, positive thought, and encouragement. It truly makes such a difference to me and to the world.

When I was a child, I felt like a stranger in a strange land. It was as if some alien stork made a wrong turn at a galaxy far, far away and dropped me on this planet called Earth. What seemed most important to others wasn't so much to me. What was important to me didn't seem important to others. Throughout the roller-coaster ride of my life experience, a huge shift has taken place. During months of meditative silence and stillness, I have experienced my own ocean of truth deeper and deeper, where boundaries of form and spirit continue to melt into one. In our humanity, we create distinctions and crave boundaries. I am human, and I long for the taste of the avocado, the feel of my feet sinking into the sand as the tide goes out, the held hand of a loved one, my own expressions in art and writing, and my solitary gaze upward into the timeless, starlit sky. Yet I remain intricately connected, soul-to-soul, with everyone. Illness beckons us to shed our protective layers and connect deeply with everyone at our very essence. Ultimately, we are not our role, our name, or our singular personality. We are not a patient, a staff member, a nurse, a doctor, the valet, the volunteer, the illness, or the cure. We all wear different garments draped over the same spirit as we learn lessons on how to live, love, and be open. The yin and yang of the whole.

In our recovery, can we remove the narrow blinders that limit us to our small self, and expand to feel our connection to everyone? Can we choose not to live imprisoned in our own individual boxes with sharp edges and defined boundaries, which we strive so diligently to decorate, in order to prove how different and separate we are? If we can shed our boundaries, we learn we aren't our box. We then come to realize that it isn't even about stepping outside the box. We finally rest in the knowledge that there *is* no box. We are all one. This is our practice as we move through and give meaning to our path of treatment and recovery. We look into the eyes and the heart of each person we meet on our journey. In connecting with each of them, we connect to a place of healing within ourselves. We are no longer contracting inward to an isolated and often "poor me" universe, to the identity of our illnesses, or to our own small selves. Instead we open outward and connect with the vastness of the sky, the strength of the trees, the entire human spirit, the infinite galaxies, and the divine. Our healing becomes everyone's healing. Everyone's healing becomes our healing.

Our lesson in life is to enjoy and appreciate our seeming separateness, while at the same time, know that we are all one. We are all born from the same energy, the same creation, and the same source, with its various names. All of us are involved in this great dance: the blossom, the chirp of the bird, and the caress of the wind. I am a part of everything and everyone. I am at once the blooming flower and the wilting petal, the rising and setting sun, the blade of grass, and ever expansive sky. I hear myself in the cricket chirping late into the summer night and the rustle of the invisible wind. I see myself in both the homeless and the rich. If we know that we are not unlike all things, while being connected to the source of all things, then all things are possible. One is all, all is one. We are not separate from life; we are life. We are not separate from each other; we are each other. When we breathe, everything breathes. In the last moments of my life, all the borders will crumble as everything blends into the oneness that has always been there. We see ourselves and each other as individual drops of water. We think we have such grandeur, might, and presence until we join the sea. Ah, then what power!

I gaze at my living and dining room as I sit on a chair up against my front door, holding the rising and falling pulleys for my physical therapy exercises above my head. Silence and this moment shift me to a parallel dimension. It is as if I have been transported into some animated movie as each object in the room seems to slowly come alive. Defined edges disappear, a name is abandoned, and seemingly inanimate objects become animate. I see and feel the memory of each person's heart, soul, sweat, and tears in every piece of furniture. I am transported backward in time. The antique hutch that belonged to my parents sits proudly in my dining room and is no longer random pieces of wood. Instead, in rapid multiple exposures, I see a tree, a lumberjack, a carpenter, the carpenter's family, a truck driver, a salesperson, and the makers of the vehicle that carried it to my parents' home over sixty years ago. I sense their anticipation and excitement as it makes its debut in their living room. Within it, I feel their love as they sit together in their first home, deciding which cherished pieces are to fill the hutch's empty shelves. I recall the countless times we all pulled open the drawers to retrieve some housed object and brought it into the light of day. I see its desk fold open to reveal treasured objects kept there while my mother sat in front of it to pay bills. I remember my mother, years later, inspired with creativity, giving it a new life by antiquing it in greens and gold. I have bittersweet memories of bringing it into my house after their deaths and feeling the company of my parents. It now sits in my living room, embedded with all the love and memories that brought it to this moment in time.

There is the baby grand piano. I see my mom receiving it in eighth grade as a graduation present. She sits before it for the first time in awe, gratitude, and excitement and gently places her hands on the keys. Her heart opens with each strike of the ebony and ivory as she gives the instrument its first breath of life. I see its movement to our first home in Arcadia and then to Whittier. Since then, how many songs has it played, how many people has it entertained, and how many melodies have wafted into eternity? How many bad notes have been struck as my sisters and I learned new songs? How many times did she sit beside us and patiently attempt to teach us to play? I remember with all my senses the countless times she played the songs of her heartthrob, Dean Martin, as the melodies made their way from a distance to my upstairs room. I remember the peace I felt inside knowing she was calm and happy. I recall our dog who always came to lie beside the pedals as she began to play. Within the piano are her words, "This will be yours someday, Suzette." My dread of losing her was combined with the stunned possibility of having this beloved instrument of hers in my home one day. I hear all the songs she composed and that have now disappeared into the mahogany. Now the piano sits in my living room and expresses great love. It is rarely played, but stands in majesty and memory of my mom. Present. Alive.

Everything is connected to all things. Everywhere I gaze, a ball of memories seems to unravel in all directions to release its spirit and love. How do we separate anything and anyone from anything or anyone? Everything is intricately stitched together. The antique television that rests in my dining room fills me with the laughter, friendship, and love that my sister and I shared when we bought it at a local antique shop. I am embraced by the joy, connection, and conversations of a trade I did with a spirited, artistic couple in return for a cherished, beautiful, and whimsically designed revolving shelf, which brings me much joy. The artwork of an interpretation of my mom at her piano as a young girl is filled with not only the talent of the artist, but my connection with his wife and their sweet children. I feel the love and generosity of my partner, now beyond the veil, who designed and built everything in my art studio to allow my creativity to flow with greater ease. In each shelf and table are his many frustrating trips to Home Depot, his precious hours plotting its design, and his love, sweat, and hard work. I revel at how it stands well-used and full of love almost twenty years later. I see pictures on the wall of my sweet kitty, Tattoo, and my dear family. They come alive with memories captured in that moment in time, but also unfold outward in all directions. I see every link in each object's chain. Nothing appears separate. Every ripple creates an endless ripple. Everything matters. Everything offers its energy, its memories, and its presence.

Sitting in my patio chair, I see all the gifts of love from my journey over the last year. I do not just hear the chimes. I feel the time searching for this gift, the generosity, the anticipated opening, the hanging, and each rustle of the wind allowing them to sing their song. Prayer flags wave in the wind with their loving, healing messages. Presents of blooming plants and flowers stand tall. My family bought bird feeders as gifts, which have attracted countless feathered friends into my life. Gifts of cat and squirrel sculptures, as well as a metal peacock of brilliant colors and feathers blowing in the wind embrace me with their loving thoughtfulness and generosity. Nearby, a beautiful custom-tile koi fish stepping stone and bird bath, which was freely given by an artist friend, remind me of his generous heart. A metal sign given to me by my sisters reads "The Journey is Everything" and hangs from umbrella to umbrella, always reminding me of my motto. A handmade piece of art glass from a dear friend sparkles with love in the sunlight. I am surrounded by so much beauty and joy. All are alive and filled with love. I am one with all. All is one.

I see the billions of unfathomable stars above the billions of blades of grass. I see each microcosmic world and also those that explode outward to the infinitely mysterious yet ordered eternity. I kneel before this vast tapestry. I'm as integral to everything and everyone as everything and everyone is to me on the planet. When you pull one tiny thread from a sweater, everything starts to unravel. We are all inseparable and equally important. We are all one silence, yet a diversity of voices. What lies within makes us one. What lies without, separates. We create the individual lyrics of our own story, but also yearn to connect to the underlying melody that binds us all. There is a deep and always reverberating chorus that is found beyond the solitary note of who we think we are. When we recognize and sing to the source within us, we are all connected as one. Great healing happens in that place of no lines where the ocean blends into the sky, where borders crumble, where I become you, and we all become the infinite. It is a place where all thoughts disappear and we all drop into the one pulse that connects all of our hearts. When we move and live in this place, the healing of our body, mind, and spirit happens naturally and effortlessly.

In the midst of our recovery in this crazy, chaotic, and you versus me world, our work in endless progress is keeping the door to our hearts open, and continuing to feel the immense healing power and beauty in our connection with everything and everyone.

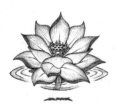

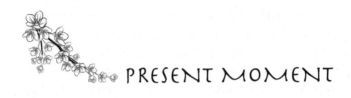

# PRESENT MOMENT

Be here now.
-Ram Dass

The present moment is the only moment available to us
... and is the door to all moments.
-Thich Nhat Hahn

At times it is as if I am waking from a dream. Another dimension. My narrow aperture broadens to a more wide angle lens. For months, I have been residing in the neck of the hourglass, moment to moment. The path I travel in my house begins to shift, not just from the bed to the bathroom, or from the bed to the patio chair. Now it begins to open in the other direction again. I see a glimpse of a former life. Ah, across my lawn is an art studio! Did I really go in there, day in and day out, to make a living with my art for twenty years? A silver Toyota is parked out back. Is that mine? Did I ever use both eyes and really drive with two healthy arms? There is a big white van in front of my house. It is filled with artwork. Did I lift and pack my entire display and artwork to travel solo across the US to fine art shows? I open my closet and the wardrobe is a distant memory. Only a few items with zip-up fronts that don't have be put over my head are used now. I see boxes labeled "Retreats" and "Workshops." Did I lead all of those? I see a framed certificate saying I am a third-degree black belt in tai chi. Did I use this body to flow through countless forms and wield weapons with "taken-for-granted" abandon? There is a framed picture of my partner Chuck and I kayaking through New Zealand. How I wish he were still alive and here to accompany me on this journey. Another picture is of "Hodnett Castle" in Ireland, which was discovered when I cashed in my life for solo adventures in travel. More and more I remember—yes.

Then a glance in the mirror catches me unaware: a distorted and paralyzed face, a missing ear, right arm in a sling, one usable eye, and skinny legs and arms. What was and what is collide at the intersection of the present moment. I pause there and greet the unfamiliar body with my very familiar spirit. New adventures await us.

We are innocent prisoners who are given 3/6/9/12 month reprieves. Going before our oncologists in structured intervals can feel as if we are going before a warden to determine if we are to be given another sentence or be set free. If it is another sentence, we never really know what we did or didn't do during those months to render the current verdict. A clear scan can feel like a huge reprieve allowing the anxiety to disappear into the vast distance of the horizon. As our next follow-up for a new scan slowly approaches, everything begins to loom larger and larger once again. It is as if we are driving toward what looks like a slight incline, and little by little, we remember all too well that it is actually a foreboding mountain. There is no turning back. The trajectory of our lives can change in an instant.

How do we get the anxiety to loosen its grip, even when it is staring us in the face? How do we soften the edge of this always approaching reality? This is true for all of us, but perhaps only those who have gone through the wilderness of diagnosis and treatment can know what it is like to be looking squarely in the eye at our seeming fate, time and time again.

The only answer is to embrace life, day by day and moment to moment. Our healing journey is our great training and immutable Zen master. The lesson continually repeats itself: Breathe and return to this present moment. Let go of all the possible fearful scenarios that rise in the mind. Just be right here and right now. Simple, but not easy. Of course, the truth is it's an illusion that we are the only ones who live under a verdict that can change in a moment's notice. Life has a very deft sleight of hand. Each day is a gift for all, with only a possible reprieve into the next. At any moment, at any hour, and on any day, anyone's life can be taken from them in the blink of an eye.

During the twists, turns, and bumpy roads of our healing path, we want to detour from the present moment in the hopes of avoiding nausea, pain, weakness, anxiety, and fatigue. If we can accept what is happening and be with just one moment in time, the here and now can actually ease our discomfort and lighten a heavy burden. In the present moment is only a single throb, one twist of the muscle, a solitary burning sensation, and an inhale and exhale. Suffering is resisting the present moment. In trying to push it away, it just returns to us stronger. We don't have to like the moment, just accept it for what is.

The magic of the present moment is that it can make all things possible. As my sisters and I "optimized" chemotherapy, it was only completed by taking it all one step and one moment at a time. Coming from treatment, it often felt like there was no way I could do the half-hour exercise walk. However, moment to moment, I reached my goal despite the exhaustion and nausea. Holding my sister's belt loop and listening to her relaxing voice, I felt her calm center and knew she wasn't in a hurry. She let me lead, pause, allow a wave to come and go, and then take a few more steps. Taking it all moment to moment, we had accomplished the half-an-hour walk. Next, I was to submerge myself in a hot bath for a half an hour. She drew the water. After only a few minutes in the tub, the heat felt suffocating and overwhelming. It seemed there was no way I could sit in there for thirty minutes. Instead, I focused on my breathing for one minute, then another. How could I drink the required eight cups of water? I couldn't, but I could take one sip at a time. Moment to moment. I looked at the rubber ducks and felt the sensation of the water opening my pores to absorb the chemo. Breathe in and out. No past, no future. Just the sweat on my brow. The deep pulse of my heart. The flush of my skin. The time is up and the cups of water are empty. I am back in bed. If I don't push away the nausea, my body relaxes and softens. I feel the warmth of clean sheets, the gentle beat of my heart, the soft breeze of my breath, and the expansive night sky. Becoming one with the present moment calms the rough waters of my mind and thus my body. Just this moment. There is nowhere to go, nothing to do. Rest and float with the waves. Don't resist the ride. Inhale, exhale.

Fast-forwarding into our future makes everything appear solid and permanent, which it never is. So much of what we think and do is born of our fear of an imagined scenario. Fear is created by our minds not being in sync with what is true right here and right now. If we can allow whatever is happening to just be, it returns to us the gift of clarity from its peace. In one moment, a neighbor's dog barks loudly, then there is a silence between the barks. The wind blows and the chimes clamor wildly. The breeze softens and the next moment is quiet.

Everything changes. Sitting in the present moment, I could truly experience what was around me. I was one with the slow dance of the changing shadows, a bird on a wire, the evening lullaby of crickets, the sound of children holding on to the last remnants of light as they play ball on the street, the rustle of a single leaf, a ray of sunshine spotlighting a glistening dew drop on a petal, and the intent of the wind before it blew. Moment to moment. Everything changes.

The quickest way to enter the present moment and connect with the aliveness, vast space, and our true inner being is through the breath. The breath was at the center of my healing. Breathing slowly and mindfully without breaking the delicate thread emptied me into infinite space. If I followed the tiniest opening, I could breathe into the discomfort, fears, grudges, history, all of the "before," and out of an imagined future and flow into the expansiveness of the now. This is the present moment, which is without time and space and is always complete, whole, perfect, and peaceful.

Is my life the same or different than the moment before my diagnosis? At this very moment, do I have a problem or does it only appear if I fast-forward into some imagined future? I may have some challenges. I have a patch on one eye, a sling on my arm, ever-changing sensations, fatigue, and a diagnosis. However, if we remain in the present, nothing becomes "solid" because moment-to-moment everything is forever shifting. If our worries, fears, and thoughts snap us out of this moment, we return to the breath and allow the present moment to be our deep healing.

Is not each moment in time a freeze frame in which, only when put together one after the other and flicked with our thumbs, we see the action created from the noun? Moment to moment, I am framed in time. Only moments from now I will be changing the picture, getting up, and going inside. Each moment dying into the next. Each one full. Each one complete. Each one an eternity into itself.

Moment to moment. Life goes on and waits for no one.

Sweet, warm embrace of an afternoon with a calming breeze entering through the screen door. Day turns to dusk. Rod Stewart sings "Moon River." There is the simple task of folding clothes ever so slowly with one hand and one eye, but somehow this moment slips deep into my soul. Precious. Transient. A gift. What is life but a series of precious moments that often go unnoticed, unappreciated, and disguised by the "to do" list while looking for the next moment rather than embracing this one?

Sometimes, like this moment that reaches into my soul and catches me unaware, so also can the diagnosis. Ah, yes, what does it all mean? Life is still unfolding moment to moment, not different in many ways but changed in others. Words have the power to free or the power to imprison. If my thoughts attach to a barrage of words that corral me into the past and future, then I am no longer living. The present moment frees us because to be there, we must be free of the antics of our mind. Then we rest in just what is: the sound of the sprinklers, the folding of a warm towel just out of the dryer, the hint of a soft breeze, a bird chirping in the distance, the bark of a dog, or the hug of a shadow from a nearby tree. Each moment unfolds into the next.

My "religious release" teacher I had as a young Catholic girl in public school would come and escort us to her home for a lesson once a week. One afternoon, three of us sat around a picnic table in her backyard. Unlike the nuns who often taught from fear, she always inspired us with her passion and sense of mystery. On this day, a kitchen timer sat in the middle of the table. She mindfully turned the timer to one minute, asked us to listen as closely as we could, and released the dial. We sat, somewhat confused but mesmerized, as the ticking of the clock seemed as connected to us as our own heartbeat. We followed each individual sound of the timer. The one minute did not sweep by, but instead seemed to last an eternity. We were not sure of the importance of the timer and its possible religious lesson, but it was clear from our teacher's quiet, focused presence that she wanted us to listen closely and completely. When the timer rang after sixty seconds, she said: "You will never have this minute back. Moment to moment you are given a choice. You can choose during each moment to be kind or cruel. You can decide to fight with your brother or sister or not. You are the artist painting your canvas of how you want the picture of your life to look. Moment to moment. It is all you have. There is no such thing as the future. The past is gone. Life is only each tick of the timer." A guru disguised as a housewife opened her house to six children once a week.

"It is not fair that this happened to you." People will say this to me. It is said out of great compassion. Yet, I truly can't be cheated out of a guarantee I never had. None of us know more than just this moment. The beauty in this journey is perhaps to remind all of us of how precious, unpredictable, and important each moment is, which is something we often overlook in the hubbub of our lives. Gifts may not always be wrapped in a tidy ribbon and a bow. Let us awaken and live deeply within each moment that is given to us. Pour ourselves into our lives. Express our love to all. Fear not. Embrace what is in front of us. Move always in the direction of our dreams. Moment to moment.

I give thanks to each individual moment-to-moment stitch of "no-time" in the great tapestry of my life over the last year.

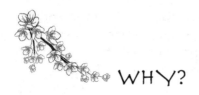

# WHY?

Only don't know.
-Seung Sahn

How did I get thee? Let me count the ways.

Many sources will offer reasons why—the Internet, books, YouTube, doctors, and well-meaning family and friends.

Choose a door: 1) physical, 2) emotional, 3) spiritual, or 4) all of above.

Thousands of research studies have explained mutated genes and chromosomes. Many point to environmental toxins and hereditary predispositions. Others blame stressful lifestyles, processed food, polluted air, wrong thinking, lack of faith, and expressed or unexpressed emotions. Did we agree to it in a previous lifetime? Is it my karma? Is it what I thought—or didn't think? Something I did or didn't do? Is it a lesson for me or for those around me to learn? Did I stray out of the vortex? Is it a message from God?

Genetic counselors seek knowledge. I spent too much time surfing as a kid without sunscreen. Translocated chromosomes 14-18 have prevented apoptosis (programmed cell death) in my DNA. Living behind an oil refinery plant for over ten years was a deep insult to my immune system. And I have a strong family history of cancer.

The gavel strikes judgment on a merry-go-round of responsible parties. I created it. No, my surroundings are responsible. Wait! What my parents ate and drank and breathed is really to blame. It is a toxic society, a poisonous world.

Am I innocent until proven guilty? Is there insufficient evidence to proclaim a verdict? The merry-go-round turns faster and faster until it all becomes a blur in the thunderous roar of diagnosis and treatment. Do we really have to strike the gavel and proclaim judgment and responsibility? There is, of course, a certain security if we know, offering us a feeling of ground beneath us as all seem to crumble. Of course, it also makes sense to want to know the answer if it means there is a possibility of finding a cure.

However, perhaps no judgment need be made on anything. As always, the infinite sees in 360°. Not me. My mind would love to figure out the who, what, when, why and how and welcomes certainty and control. My heart knows that the frenzy of the mind isn't where peace, truth, higher wisdom, and healing reside.

I have let go of any need to know. I rest in not knowing. I surrender to the reality that I ultimately don't know anything. Scientists who spend millions on research don't know. The Internet is full of conflicting research, testimonials, and possibilities. This doesn't mean not to look at how I can improve my health, diet, and immune system. No matter what is happening in any of our lives, it is important to take our own personal inventory of responsibility. What negative thoughts and stresses do we allow in our lives? Are we emotionally happy and spiritually alive? Are our lives sung in a frenzied melody or peaceful cadence with continual crescendos of joy? These are the questions we must ask ourselves, illness or no illness.

However, it is not for us to ask why, but instead to bring meaning to whatever is placed in our path and make each moment of our life sacred. Otherwise it is easy to fall victim to feelings of guilt, blame, and overwhelming confusion. When going through the onslaught of treatment, we do not need to be trying to figure our why this diagnosis has fallen into our laps. Instead we must rest in not knowing and accept our unfolding path. In emptying ourselves of our need to know, we can then rest in peace instead of the frenzy of our mind.

To me, what is most important is that I meet every circumstance with a spirit of acceptance and an open heart. I must continue to say yes to the experience, remaining open to all the healing energy and love that surrounds me. If I need to ask "why," then it is also a slippery slope to asking "why me?" This question can lead to bitterness, confusion, resentment, anger, and despair. Our mind can then run a marathon of all the countless scenarios of "why this" and "why that" and all the reasons that our life "isn't fair." Let us make the question not "why" as we move through this journey but "why not?"

Why not us to have this challenge as much as anyone else?

Why not embrace what rests in our lap, right here and right now, rather than look to some imagined, better future?

Why not bring love, acceptance, peace, and hope into our diagnosis and recovery rather than bitterness, anger, resentment, and despair?

Why not focus on our blessings as we travel the healing path instead of sinking into the sad story of the illness?

Why not move forward in trust instead of fear?

Why not let go of our need to know and embrace our "don't know" mind, say yes, and trust that everything is here to teach us?

There are many different types of healing along our journey: our spirit, body, mind, and our relationships with others and the divine. What is most important is that whatever seeming obstacles we have on our path, we don't have to figure out why but instead continue to learn, love, and be joyful. In the state of not knowing, there is infinite space for everything. We can then rest in the miraculous nature of our world.

So here is to letting go of all the "whys" and allowing the mind to drop deeply into the wide embrace of our hearts, the home of deep healing.

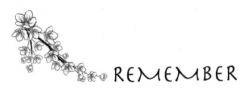

# REMEMBER

*Promise me you'll always remember: You're braver than you believe,*
*and stronger than you seem, and smarter than you think.*
-A. A. Milne

We experience something deeply. However it is often easy in the clutter, clamor, and humanness of our lives to forget. It takes a great deal of love to remember and keep something alive in the midst of its seeming absence. It has to burn a space deep in our hearts and find its place on the altar of our own sacred passions and people. How easy is it to forget in all walks of life? Our friends we once vowed always to remember, loved ones who pass on while we remain, and experiences that change us, the air of importance now taken out of them like a deflated balloon. How easy it is to even forget our own relationship with the infinite, amid the hubbub we create for ourselves.

Stripped naked during our treatment and recovery and then moving back into the world, it is perhaps not so desirable for us to deeply remember. Many of us don't want to return to that wilderness. Yet this is the place where we are most vulnerable and connected to the breath, stillness, and knowing. It is a place of truth.

Our days in the wilderness of our healing are not times to be buried and forgotten, no matter the outcome. Instead, they are times to be remembered and honored. They are not to be remembered in order to retell the story, again and again, but to allow our triumphs to buoy us through each unfolding chapter to come. In remembering, we bring life and meaning to our journey, as well as love and gratitude to all those we met along the path. I will always remember the tender, selfless love of my family, the deep kindness, compassion, and generosity of Team Suzette, baby steps turned into leaps, visions fulfilled, the expertise and compassion of my doctors, and the miracle of my healing. I seek to remember all the gifts so I can then return them to the world.

The journey has been everything. As with anything, how our lives are going to unfold is always a mystery, an unknown. The wheel of my life skidded in a sharp turn. I could barely move. I was dependent on others, embracing life tenderly, tenuously, moment to moment, and breath to breath after a fourteen-hour surgery, months of radiation, chemotherapy, physical therapy, and more surgeries. However, I do not remember this journey for its illness and insults. It has been a year of faith, triumphs, blessings, generosity, friendship, and expansive acts of kindness. I remember and see a beautiful, amazing tapestry woven together with golden threads of love. I may not be what was, but I am amazed at what is. I see a testimony to the body's amazing capacity to heal, and also the spirit's incredible power to uplift and persevere. I see a body that may be different, but it is learning new steps to best dance with my ever-changing energy, sensations, and flow. If I cling to wanting what was, I will suffer. Freedom resides in accepting, adapting, and learning from what falls on my path. I continue to have a life abundant with great blessings, deep faith, and unfolding opportunities. I seek to always remember the gifts given without consideration and with immense grace.

All of us need to remember how far we have come. We must remember how we were willing to show up like valiant warriors, again and again, to face the insults and assaults of treatment and keep riding toward the sunset. We need to remember so we can continue to draw strength, resiliency, and courage from our journey. We shall remember how despair becomes hope, how illness becomes health, how much love heals, and how kindness lifts the spirit. We must remember the journey and how it stripped us to our beautiful core to allow our spirits to shine through, so we could know ourselves at a deeper and deeper level. No matter what the challenge, it is always healthy to remember how far we have traveled down the winding and often bumpy road of our lives.

Then and now? It amazes and inspires me to remember how far I have come.

Then: A missing ear.
Now: Still missing, but doing a great comb-over.

Then: Right arm in a sling for six months and limited movement from a severed spinal accessory nerve.
Now: Doing tai chi and my art.

Then: Eye covered in a patch for ten months.
Now: A skin graft and here's looking at you with two eyes!

Then: After surgery, some unwelcome visitors remaining.
Now: All kicked to the far side of the moon.

Then: Couldn't move my head left to right.
Now: Short drives in my car.

Then: A tiny opening for pureed baby food.
Now: Chewing with more food going down the hatch.

Then: Unable to make it to our dojo retreat at Mt. Baldy last year.
Now: My body and my spirit soared up the mountain to train this year.

Then: Couldn't hold a pair of scissors in my hand.
Now: Created the 5.5′ × 4.5′ 3D mixed media art piece entitled *The Journey is Everything.*

Then: Couldn't sleep more than ten minutes.
Now: Getting more and more beauty sleep.

Then: In a hospital bed.
Now: Sleeping in my futon bed.

Then: Cards read to me.
Now: Reading to myself.

Then: Practicing tai chi through just the breath.
Now: Received my fourth-degree black sash and teaching again.

Then: Couldn't lift a paper cup with a little water.
Now: Can lift a one-pound weight with my compromised right arm.

Then: Unable to shower.
Now: Soaking in bubble baths.

Then: Sitting in the garden dictating a message to Team Suzette .
Now: Sitting at my garden patio desk in a chair, typing the updates myself.

Then: Unable to cook for myself.
Now: Making a mean organic chicken and vegetable soup.

Then: Face in the mirror looking like a strange visitor from a strange planet.
Now: Face in the mirror looking more like an old friend.

And some things remain:

Then: Spirit strong.
Now: Spirit strong.

Then: The deep love and support of Team Suzette family and friends.
Now: The deep love and support of Team Suzette family and friends.

Then: Moment to moment, breath to breath living.
Now: Moment to moment, breath to breath living.

Then: Appreciating each day.
Now: Appreciating each day.

Perhaps most importantly, we must remember who we truly are. We are not our petty resentments, fears, and guilts. No matter what is happening in our bodies, we are whole and perfect. We have divine purpose in being here and are an intricate and sacred thread on the tapestry of life.

When we return to the hubbub of a life of distractions and clutter, it is easy to forget our journey. In the stillness of recovery we have shed our armor and moved closer and closer to the light. Let us not return to our protective layers, useless thoughts, and insignificant concerns, but continue to connect with life in an embrace of the heart.

I do not want stillness, silence, and connection with nature and the divine to become memories tucked away in a drawer, but realities to be lived with, fed upon, and breathed into every day. I want to remember all the precious gifts received, so I can return them to the world in an endless circle of giving and receiving love. No matter what the terrain before us, we must remember to keep the faith, stay strong, trust the bigger picture, and reach out in love and gratitude to all we meet.

If we keep remembering, it will lead us to remember everything. Why we are here. That we are not alone. That we are connected to everyone and everything. That we are loved. That we are love.

Let us not forget our journey, whatever it is and wherever it takes us. Let the golden threads of love that have woven our healing path together catch the sunlight and continue to illuminate the road before us.

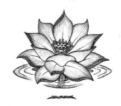

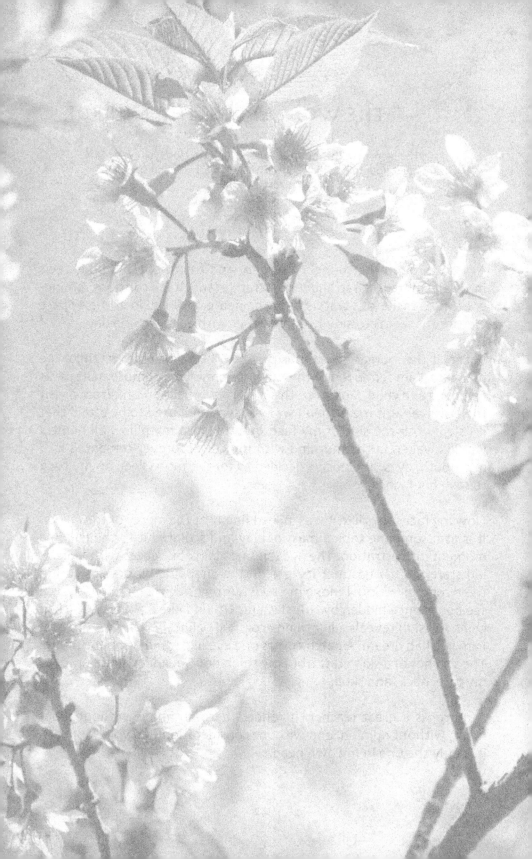

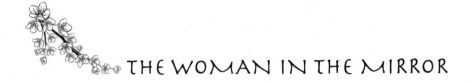

# THE WOMAN IN THE MIRROR

The woman in the mirror is a grand illusion. Close your eyes,
quiet your mind, and connect with the vastness and spirit of
who you truly are.

It's only forms that change, not essence.
Ram Dass

As I go through the tunnel of surgery and treatment, my body feels more and more like a stranger in a strange land. It is a constant reminder of the treacherous waters I now navigate. Like Hal in *2001: A Space Odyssey*, it seems to slowly deconstruct with each passing day.

I gaze at the woman in the mirror. She still startles me, catching me unaware. I am reminded of the fun house mirrors in amusement parks I enjoyed as a child. However, this distorted reflection isn't from a visit to a carnival; it is me. When I was very young, I used to be afraid that if I slept with the side of my face smashed into my pillow all night, I would awaken in the morning with my cheek forever cemented into my mouth, eyes, and nose. I decided to forevermore sleep on my back to save my face.

Now my face looks like it was indeed finally at the mercy of the pillow. It is as if someone took a mass of clay and sculpted it to the left in a moment of frustration. The eye does not blink but gazes with a piercing stare. An ear has met its fate on the chopping block. Lips curl in the wrong direction. I move my face but one side rebels in paralysis. I see bones once hidden by soft flesh protruding like a poverty-stricken child. My skin reveals a lightning-scorched oak tree. Hair falls out as if I am in a bad dream. A patch covers one eye like some wannabe pirate. The stitches of a skin graft from my thigh now meander aimlessly over my face, neck, and skull.

A mirror is a great teacher. It reflects back an image without judgment, without opinion, and without consideration. If a voice appears, it is only the one in my own head.

It is wise for all of us to bow before our mirror. What do we see when we gaze at the image reflected back at us? "Oh no! When did those gray strands appear?" "Ugh, I spot a pimple." "What? I'm losing my hair!" "There is my dad's hooked nose." "I need to lose weight!" We define what we see in the mirror as ourselves. This is the portrait we cling to and both want to change and not ever have change. This is the fate that befalls many of us. We look in the mirror and see what we don't like, what we wish to change, and the relentless passage of time. We see the droop of an eye, a blemish on the skin, or a wrinkle from too many years on our journey. We do not look and give thanks for the beauty and miracle we are: the eyes that allow us to see the rise of the morning sun, ears to listen to a symphony of birds, nose to inhale and exhale to keep us alive, a mouth to taste a smörgåsbord of delicacies, and skin that miraculously holds our insides in a soft container.

I shut my eyes and the curtain closes on my image. "Ha! I still feel myself here!" As the image in the mirror fades more deeply into blackness, I feel more and more truly me. "Ah, this is me!" I open an eye. The partially distorted image reappears. "Ha! Well, who is that then?" I close my eyes once again leaving this image behind. I let myself reside in this feeling of "always was and always will be." The darkness from my closed eyes somehow reveals my ever-present light inside.

I am indeed the constant, unchanged soul. However, I am also this body. Resentment and bitterness toward my body could easily take the place of love and affection. It would be so easy to focus on and long for what was instead of embracing what is. Our natural tendency is to step outside of our body in an effort to escape both its emotional and physical pain. Yet, it is so important for me to instead see and appreciate it for its amazing job of deep healing, despite the constant insults of being poisoned, nuked, and carved. We must continually remind ourselves that our energy is being used to heal, and our bodies are indeed strong. Everything goes inward to rebuild, but will later expand outward to align with our spirit.

I look again in the mirror and stare at my image. I explore its new twists and turns, which tell the unfolding story of my journey. I admire its strength and resiliency, as it has risen above all to continue to heal me. I send love deep into every cell. When I chose not to have surgery when new "unwelcome guests" appeared during radiation, it continued in its perfect healing to kick all to the far side of the moon.

I respect my body. It underwent a fourteen-hour surgery and came up standing, not unlike the inflatable clown with a weighted bottom that I would punch as a child, only for it to return upright with a smile on its face. I appreciate my body for taking endless drips of chemotherapy and the burn of radiation while continuing to heal. I love this body that pulled me like a mule horse out to City of Hope each day. I admire how it peeked out to the world with one eye covered in a patch, still connected with all. I cherish this body with its distorted and paralyzed face, tethered neck, drooping shoulder, and embroidered face from a large skin graft. I honor my body which continues to expand outward to the world, giving "hugs" hand-to-hand, and connected at the heart. I marvel at how my left hand learned how to write and maneuver when my right arm was in a sling. I even love the missing ear, which allows me to listen more fully to the world. I say "welcome" to the narrow opening that is my mouth, which now makes me slow down, one tiny bite at a time, as I taste each morsel more completely. I love this body for all the places that remain unchanged and spacious enough to absorb the ever-changing sensations, as well as the merry-go-round of symptoms that I now use as a reminder of the miracle of being alive. It is important for me to keep loving this ever-changing form and soften around the hard edge of its appearance, so it can be free to heal deeply and completely. I am so grateful for my body, which exceeds all expectations, knows not the meaning of limitation, and is a tangible testimony to the miracle of my healing.

I vow to love it as it has loved me, to persevere as my body has continued to persevere, and to remember that it is my best friend who has been triumphant over pain, poisons, and excavation. It loves me as I seek to love it. What I see in the mirror is a testimony to the miracle of my healing.

Throughout our journey, we need to listen to our body and treat it with respect and appreciation. It is our best friend. It may feel like we want to rid ourselves of the pain, anxiety, and fear within our body. We may be angry at it as it weakens and changes. These are all more reasons to stay open and loving. We must give our body powerful messages of compassion and tenderness, commending it on its awesome job of healing us deeply. We must find a space of comfort within it and expand outward, trusting that moment to moment, all is healing.

I look in the mirror. I smile and look at my right side, then, while still smiling, the left side of my face. These are two very different sides of me. From my left you see a distorted, paralyzed face with no seeming smile and a missing ear. If you gaze at my right side, you will see a smile and my former face. Suzette: the same or different?

Which is me? Am I my form or my endless spirit? As they say in Zen, form is emptiness and emptiness is form.

Those who practice tai chi know it is not really our "form" (movements), but what holds the form together (the breath, balance, calm, inner peace, connection to heaven and earth, and our own center) that is the most important part of our practice. So it is not so important if someone looks at me from the left or from the right; my spirit remains the same. As we say in tai chi, I am carrying an "inner smile."

The loss of anything creates grieving. A farewell. A letting go. I look at pictures of older family portraits and see my face smiling back at me. I look at the photos post-surgery and that face is gone, never to return again. Mine has changed in one fourteen-hour surgery. No one will gaze upon that form again. Each person that now meets me will see this distorted face, listen to me through forced speech, connect with me through my one piercing, non-blinking eye, and a missing ear. Ultimately, it is as if I am saying good-bye to my most cherished piece of clothing. This garment is now tailored by circumstance and the mysterious unfolding of life. It had been taken for granted in its comfort and ease. Now I must say farewell to this close, familiar friend. How would it feel to have one more day with both sides of my face tipped in a smile? Both eyes blinking? Both ears? The embroidery gone and my skin a smooth canvas? The photos are a stark reminder of what was. The face in the mirror is a clear reflection of what is. Everything changes, whether it is from a fourteen-hour surgery or the unfolding of time. With a flutter in my heart, I know that I am not this form, but an eternal soul connected with everyone and everything on this wonderful roller coaster ride of life.

I return to teach my first tai chi class out of the dojo at a local community center. A group of new students arrive who have never seen or known me before the surgery. What will they think of this teacher, who has a distorted, paralyzed face, talks funny, is missing an ear, and has minimal motion in one arm from a severed spinal accessory nerve? I feel the challenge of connecting with this new form of me with new people. I know that it is the deeper me who teaches, but I recognize that the first connection with many can be from the snapshot they take of me with their eyes. I teach forms and movements that will have to be adapted to share with others, but what I am always truly teaching in tai chi is stillness, balance, breathing, calm, and opening the body, mind, and spirit to the world. In truth, I teach the formless behind the form. My own healing has been a marathon training in formless tai chi. In a world driven by outer beauty, appearance, and "normal," will people be able to look beyond my form? Will this new body and my timeless spirit combine to ignite interest and bring them to a deeper understanding of tai chi? I am humbled that all return after the first class.

My work is being judged for an art show. I begin chatting with an artist acquaintance I haven't seen in several years. She is startled when she finally realizes who I am and says, "Wow, I wouldn't have recognized you if you hadn't told me who you were." Ouch.

Months later, I'm at the opening night of the art show. I mention to my friend that a fellow artist on jury day said to me: "I wouldn't even recognize you if I wasn't told it was you." To be honest, there was a part of me that wanted her to respond with, "That's crazy. You don't look that different! How could she not recognize you?" Instead she said, "Some people are just honest." Ouch.

They are right. I am at a restaurant with my family. Across the table, behind the booth, is a long row of mirrors with the reflection of my face. I don't recognize the paralyzed, stoic, and distorted image that stares back at me. I am so connected to the feel of my spirit that my form can still catch me unaware in a new photo, or an unexpected glance in the mirror.

I feel its changed shape in the twists of the muscles, hardened scar tissue, challenge in talking, and missing ear, but am so connected to the me beyond the form. Out of curiosity, I load a picture of my "old face" in the "Faces" option in my iPhoto on my computer. It then scans five thousand pictures in my library and brings up hundreds of photos with me in them. When I choose my "new face" it searches long and hard, but doesn't recognize the changed form in any of the pictures. I guess they don't have the technology to capture my spirit yet, which remains the same.

Thank you to those who said they didn't see my face because my spirit shone through so brightly. Thank you to those who, in their own honesty, said they wouldn't know me now if they weren't told who I was. I have learned from both. In the sting of the words from the people who didn't recognize my new face, I am reminded that there is still a part of me attached to my form. The reality of what is now and how others see me is still able to, in certain moments, jam my gears. The kind words of the others remind me of who I truly am, and that my connection with the world is heart-to-heart, not face-to-face.

I slip into the warm embrace of the bath water and bubbles caress me. I explore my body like a new lover. The soap slides into my hand and I create a thick lather. I am an infant having a bath for the first time, being held in the protective arms of their mother. I explore this new body. I touch my face and its changed contours. I discover bumpy hills that were once flat, rolling plains. Bones in my neck and shoulders protrude, like guy-lines to support the new freestanding structure resulting from a severed spinal accessory nerve. I find the space where an ear no longer resides, but instead the odd and unfamiliar skin of my thigh. I follow the twists, turns, and crevasses of this new terrain of the graft on my face, neck, and skull. I reach out and slide the soap along each arm and leg. I gently hold each bony limb and assure them they will once again be covered by a bigger buffer of flesh. For perhaps the first time, I experience this changed body on both a deeply physical and emotional level. I offer my body appreciation for staying strong even though it is thinner. I love it for all it can still do. I revel at its strength despite the insults and injuries of treatment and surgery. A solitary tear finds its way down my cheek. Is it mourning the loss of the old body, or is it moved in appreciation for this new surviving Suzette? Perhaps both.

I rinse each part of my body and step out of the tub for a slow, dry cycle with a soft bamboo towel. I feel refreshed, rejuvenated, loved, appreciated, alive, and connected to every skinny bone in my body. I say, "Thank you! You've done an amazing job!"

To be honest, sometimes I long to talk to people without them staring at the disfigurement. It is not that I care if they happen to think I am ugly, or if they are startled by my face. I understand. At times, I just long for the freedom of taking a morning walk and greeting a passerby with both sides of my mouth beaming into a great smile. To connect without their initial response of wondering, looking, feeling sorry, or not knowing what to say. For a moment, I wish they could see what was instead of what is. However, it is a fleeting moment swallowed up by an immense sky of gratitude for the miracle of my healing and the deep knowledge of who I truly am.

Sitting in silence, moment to moment, form blends to spirit and back again. When all is stripped away, what remains is not the paralyzed face, missing ear, patched eye, or an embroidered graft. Not the side effects from the chemotherapy, the burn of the radiation, or the tugging, pulling, and twisting from a severed spinal accessory nerve. Underneath is my infinite spirit, true and eternal, untouched by the parade that passes before me.

We all wear our garments. We have our Sunday best, our slick and sexy night-out clothes, and our birthday suits from the day we were born. As our body weakens, our "outer clothing" fades and we often sink more and more into our infinite spirit. We begin to remember who we truly are. Our bodies may be our beloved garments, but they are not us. We love them, tend to them, feed them, protect them, and even purify them as our temple. Yet, no matter how much we try to have them last as long as possible, what remains in the end is not this garment but the light that has always been shining within us. Everything changes except the part of us that never changes.

My body is a great vehicle. It has pedaled the Swiss Alps, backpacked through New Zealand, taken me to a fourth-degree black sash in tai chi, merged me into sexual bliss, body-surfed to exhaustion, and allowed me to hike up craggy mountain peaks.

Yet, from illness or unfolding age, our form continues to change. I grow older. I look down and see my mother's hands. Mine are now full of bulging veins, reminiscent of the relief maps I made as a child in elementary school. Brown spots have come to visit and remain. Little crevasses line my skin like a parched lizard. Because of surgery, I have a paralyzed face. An ear remains MIA. An eye does not blink and stares knowingly back at me. The burn of radiation leaves scarring behind as its calling card. Although at times it has been challenging to feel amid an onslaught of shooting nerves, burning, twisting, and spasms, the essence of me always remains untouched. Our bodies may seem to be betraying us, but never our spirit. Each of us, no matter our physical forms, are beautiful, eternal souls here to learn lessons in how to love, live, and be open.

We live in both a world of form and spirit, humanity and spirituality. Free-falling into spirit asks us to let go of what we think we are and return home to what we truly are. The form-to-spirit experience can be the gift of our healing. We return to form having tasted the depths of spirit. That knowledge is the well we draw from while also reveling in the wonders of the gift of our human form. All we are given, each experience, each pain, every sorrow, along with wonder, awe, and beauty, is our human experience that allows us to continually deepen our spiritual path.

Our very human body is our armor and protective garment. Slowly shedding it is the unfolding of our lives. Challenges ask us to let go of what we have held so dear and true. Snakes shed their skin to allow for future growth when it no longer fits the contour of their body. When they're ready to shed the old layer, they create a rip in the old skin. They often do this by rubbing against a rough, hard object, such as a rock or a log. Our life circumstances are our rocks that create a rip in us up against challenges of all kinds. We can choose to keep opening and shed what is not essential so we can create anew. If we do, we keep shedding our human form with all of its regrets, fears, ego, wanting, desiring, comparing, and judging, until our spirit is free to eternally shine. In the wilderness and stillness of my healing, I danced with spirit. The energy of the trees, the birds, and the sky were one with me. In the cosmic dance of the universe, we are all one pulsating energy. We are all a myriad of ever-changing forms, but each with brilliant rays of the same infinite and eternal source. In meditative stillness and silence, I was the blank canvas without name, identity, and form. Then from the formless I returned to form, feeling more deeply connected to my spirit.

From the squirm of the infant, to the exuberance of the child, to the grown adult, to the feeble elder, our form is ever-changing. Whether the changes are subtle from our natural aging, or monumental from illness or injury, our continual challenge is to use our physical challenges to return us to our true selves. Let the changing forms or weakness of our bodies serve to remind us that we are the strength of our soaring spirit. Once we dive deep into this eternal spirit, we will connect with the vast, empty space at the seat of all healing. Perhaps the props and circumstances of my outside life differ now, but inside I remain the same. Grateful for what I have, I live moment to moment, loving, laughing, and letting life move through me.

The woman in the mirror is a grand illusion. Close your eyes, quiet your mind, and connect with the vastness and spirit of who you truly are.

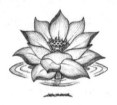

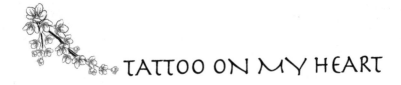

# TATTOO ON MY HEART

Love knows no boundaries between species.

I've lived with a lot of Zen masters. Most of them cats.
-Eckhart Tolle

Until we know the love of an animal,
a part of our soul is unawakened.
-Anatole France

I've been through the peaks and valleys of life and learned many lessons during both the detours and open highways on my path. But
a little hairless kitty named Tattoo shook my world, took me on an
unsuspected ride, and in many ways, prepared me for my journey
of healing. Teachers come in all shapes, sizes, and species, with and
without hair, but this seven-pound soul embodied in a Sphynx cat has
been my greatest teacher in embracing pain and illness with peace,
courage, calm, and love. Throughout all her health challenges (hypertrophic cardiomyopathy, auto-immune disease, seizures, congestive
heart failure, liver disease), her sweet disposition, healing energy to
all around her, and loving spirit remained constant.

Little Miss Tattoo let me experience the healing spirit of unconditional love, the true meaning of being in the present moment, and how to
relax into deeper and deeper places. She taught me to always expect
a miracle, and also to be the miracle itself. Her message was to not
assume or attach myself to any prediction, to let go of all fear, and
to stay open to healing. She amazed doctors with her comebacks and
never ceased to astound me with miracle after miracle in her more
than nine lives.

It is said we are given what we need and not necessarily what we
think we want. Tattoo was my gift from the divine, whose special
sweet spirit, healing energy, and unconditional love blessed me
with a deeper experience of joy, love, peace, and the power of the
present moment. I carried her many life lessons with me each day
throughout my recovery when she was no longer here in form, but
ever-present in spirit. Her body gave way to heart failure from her

hypertrophic cardiomyopathy, just days before my second diagnosis was made and I was swept into the tide of surgery and treatment. It was divine timing, as I could no longer tend to her. Now her sweet spirit could accompany me every moment, everywhere. I was no longer watching over her. She was now watching over me.

If we are willing to receive their gifts, these masters of being will crack us open to allow more of our divine light to shine. They will slow us down to see more clearly. They can soften us so that our hearts open wider. Their presence asks us to reach outside of ourselves so we can fully be ourselves. They can take us away from before and after, so we can be in the now. If we are willing to receive their gifts, these masters of being will unconditionally love us, showing us how to love ourselves and others without judgment. Their centered being relaxes us so we know the feeling of our bodies connecting more deeply to our spirit. They beckon us to flow from the visible to the invisible. They will lead us to trust in the unknown as much or more than the known. They will teach us how "to be" instead of how "to do" as their gentle souls lead us to listen inward, rather than focus outward.

Why do we have such a deep, ever-present, long-lasting, and eternal love with our animal companions? Our beloved animals are a safe haven to open up and a soft place to fall. Their love heals our body, mind, and spirit. Our relationship with them is not scarred from painful fights, hurtful words, judgments, or grievances held that compromise our love. They don't wound our egos, frustrate our spirits, or hurt our hearts. Their love is pure and freely given, knowing no space or time. Love is that place inside of complete openness and lack of judgment. Perhaps it is a place in our hearts that only an animal can reach. Many others may take residence in our hearts, but there is a special place carved out for these masters of being.

After a long day of life, with all its sometimes complexities and frustrations, Tattoo would always be there as a solid rock of love and devotion. I never had to worry about saying the wrong thing to her. She would greet me each day with such excitement and anticipation. She gave me the space to be next to her, even though she didn't feel well. She sat by my side and loved me throughout everything, with absolutely no judgment, allowing for an emptiness to let me be however I was in the present moment. That is love. How many people can give us this? The countless pills and trips to the vet may have been outside realities to help support her body, but it was the love between us that truly healed, just as each card, each message, each doorstop delivery, each contribution, and every loving intention from Team Suzette continued to heal me to a deeper and deeper level.

Tattoo showed constant courage and calm in the face of all her health challenges. She taught me how much our minds cause our suffering by defining our experience through words that we stamp as good or bad. During her unpredictable seizures, breathing challenges from an enlarging heart, immune system breakdown, and growing lymph nodes, she was not lost in worry and judgment like us humans. When she was able, she still found great joy in the simple pleasures of chasing a bug, rubbing her face against mine, curling up under my shirt, the flight of the birds outside, and the gift of a treat. Even in the midst of her pain, she remained in seemingly great gratitude for every moment with me. That doesn't mean she didn't experience bodily discomfort. However, she continually let it all go, time and time again. Her pain wasn't a foreboding shadow that followed her through each step of her journey. She didn't complain. She wasn't too thrilled about getting in the cat carrier to go to the vet, but her sweet disposition was the constant thread weaving itself throughout the journey of her illness. She continued to find great joy, experience peace in the present moment, and give and receive deep, abiding love.

What was healing for Tattoo was healing for me as well. I now more fully understand not wanting to get into a car and being driven off to a hospital where you know you will be poked and prodded, even if it eventually helps. I deeply know the feeling of a body exhausted and just in want of rest. Yes, it seemed like she "needed" to be dragged off to the vets, time and time again, especially during the last six months of her illness. Yet her weakened body really just wanted to curl up with me in peace and connection. I was always weighing the stress of the ride and the visit to the vet versus how much it could help her. Just as often, I wondered what was more healing for me: being shuttled off to the hospital day in and day out for treatment or staying home to rest and heal deeply from moment to moment.

Tattoo's greatest life lesson was to continually ask me to sink deeper and deeper into the experience of the beauty and peace of the present moment. Despite all my training in tai chi, meditation, and relaxation, it was this little hairless Zen master resting heavily on my chest in abiding, unconditional love who always reminded me to keep breathing into just this moment. We seem to only allow ourselves to "be" with our animals for short snippets of time. Then our mind tugs us back into what we "have" to do and where we "have" to go. We are often writing our "to do" list as we pet our animal. The deeper into relaxation we allow ourselves to sink with them sometimes the more insistent is the tug we feel to return to the hustle and bustle of life. Yet if we allow ourselves to open to their peace, our animals can indeed be our great teachers who calm our minds, our breathing, and offer us their stillness so we can connect with the present moment.

We always feel that there is so much that we "have to do," but when Tattoo was curled up on top of my chest, I sank deeply into just that moment. I felt like all could be postponed for hours, days, or indefinitely, and it would figure itself out. That was always the deeper truth. When she was first diagnosed with congestive heart failure, I monitored her heartbeat as she remained on my chest for days. My "to-do" list lost all meaning. Only each beat of her heart mattered. When she triumphed over the crisis, there ended up being no catastrophe that came from putting all aside. Instead, many of the items that seemed important were now inconsequential.

I so dreaded the thought of losing Tattoo to an untimely and premature death from heart failure that it was sometimes difficult to relax into the present moment with her and not allow the dark clouds of her imagined future scenarios to hover over us. My fears would invariably break the delicate thread of deep connection, the present moment, and relaxation between us. As she curled up heavily and relaxed on my chest, my training would then be to catch the projection screen of my mind whenever it flashed thoughts of her no longer with me. Then, as in any meditation, I would keep returning to the breath and the beauty of the present moment, which connected us in unconditional love. Through the breath, our divine, eternal spirits could connect without time, space, or condition. However, I would invariably break the thread by a thought or movement. If my mind would allow it, one conscious breath would return us to the present moment of love, healing, and peace.

Looking back, I spent far too much time fretting about how much time was left in the hourglass with her. I wish I could have each of those moments back to hold her lovingly in the depth of the present moment. Her living in the beauty of the here and now always reminded me to keep returning to just this moment, where all living takes place. No matter what was happening in her body, she would always just rest, right here and right now, heavily on my chest. Life, hers and mine, was always an unknown except within each precious moment in time.

This is a great reminder that all we ever have and all we can ever truly know is just this moment. This is a lesson for everyone, especially those going through the trajectory of diagnosis, treatment, and recovery. How often do we fast-forward into our future, robbing us of the precious present moment in time before us? What if chemo doesn't work? How long will I be here? What if I die? Each of our futures, hers and mine, were always a big "don't know." When we find ourselves caught up in the "what ifs" that propel us into the future, let us not miss the beauty that is right before us, lest we look back and wish that we could now have all those precious moments back when we were lost in worry. May we always remember that life is nowhere else than right before us.

Allow your animal companion to be your soft place to fall as you go through the wilderness of recovery. Let them hold you in the embrace of the present moment as they sink their being into yours. Feel their relaxation deep in your own bones. Let the vast unconditional love they offer freely saturate every cell. Experience their lack of attachment to how you look or feel as they find joy in just being close to you. Let your heart become light as you watch them play. As you open up to all the gifts they have to offer, you are also opening up to deep healing and peace. If your animal companion is no longer here, remember and connect with their loving spirit. My sweet angel Tattoo has been with me every step of my journey. I gaze at my favorite photo of the two of us. We both no longer have the same physical form. Her body is now ashes in a small container and mine is not the once familiar face in the picture. However, we are connected as we always have been: heart to heart, unconditional love to unconditional love, spirit to spirit, and soul to soul. Even though the feel of her warm, soft skin and her sweet, precious face was soothing and comforting, it was her gentleness, her peace, her healing energy, and unconditional love that was the true connection. This surrounds me forever.

We have many teachers along our path of recovery and they come in many disguises. Bow before your animal companion. They are our unfailing friends and masters in all things healing during our journey. Love heals. Unconditional love knows no illness, space, time, or species.

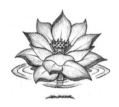

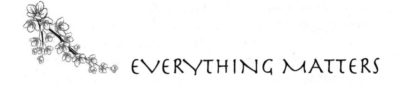

# EVERYTHING MATTERS

*He who has a why to live for can bear with almost any how.*
*-Victor Frankl*

Everything matters: each intention, each thought, every word we choose, and each step of our journey.

It matters how we greet each new day and how we say good night. It matters what we think in the dark of the wee hours. It matters what we say to ourselves when no one is listening.

It matters that we give thanks. It matters that we appreciate each gift we receive each day, however small. It matters that we give gifts every day, however small. It matters that we notice how much grace is in our lives.

It matters that we continue to care and continue to dare. It matters that we are here and each of us is a shining star in this brilliant, mysterious, and miraculous constellation. It matters that we know we are all threads connected to everything and everyone in the magnificent tapestry of life.

It matters that we have hope. It matters that we expect miracles.

It matters that we understand that cancer is another way to catapult us into experiencing the gift of our lives. It matters that we don't identify with our illness, but with our spirit. It matters that we leave "the story" behind.

It matters that we don't cling to the drama and the mind's dance around our diagnosis and prognosis. It matters that we see each other not as patients and doctors/nurses, but as fellow travelers on this journey of life.

It matters that we realize that cancer is just a word because at any moment we are healed.

It matters that we have been given the gift of life. It matters that we then believe each moment is sacred. It matters that we hold each leaf, each animal, and each other in reverence.

It matters that we keep our hearts open. It matters that we are an endless circle of giving and receiving healing love. It matters that we realize that each moment is yet another choice to choose love.

It matters that we trust the bigger picture and also what is right in front of us. It matters that we forgive and allow ourselves to be forgiven.

It matters that we keep the faith, whatever that is for us. It matters that we surrender and it matters that we believe. It matters that no matter the darkness, we keep moving toward the light and our divine purpose.

It matters that we continue to express joy.

Everything matters because everything we do and everything we say creates who we are and who we become. Everything matters because every thought and action flows outward to change the current of the universe.

It matters that we smile at the nurse taking our blood. It matters in the greetings we give to each valet, receptionist, assistant, therapist, and doctor.

It matters what we say to ourselves when we are entering the radiation tunnel. It matters what we think as the chemotherapy drips into our system.

Each baby step in our healing matters.

It matters that we keep loving our bodies and respecting them for their deep healing. It matters what we choose to eat and drink. It matters that we trust that all will be well.

It matters that we remember that we aren't only our body but also our eternal spirit.

It matters that we are grateful for each moment despite how tired, ill, or saddened we might feel. It matters that we know this too shall pass.

It matters that we help a stranger. It matters that we look heart-to-heart into the eyes of the beggar, even if we give them no money. It matters that we know we are connected to the homeless, soul-to-soul.

Each time we open our hearts and ripple outward matters. Each time we close down and stop the ripple matters.

Every magical, mystical, and miraculous breath matters.

It matters that we are here, right here and right now.

Everything matters.

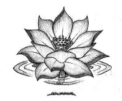

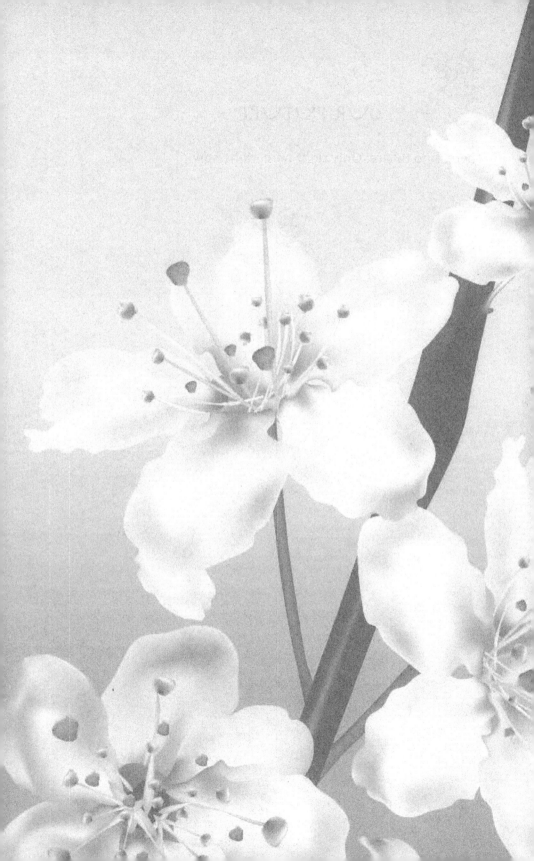

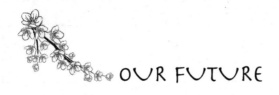

# OUR FUTURE

There is no future. Only right here, right now.

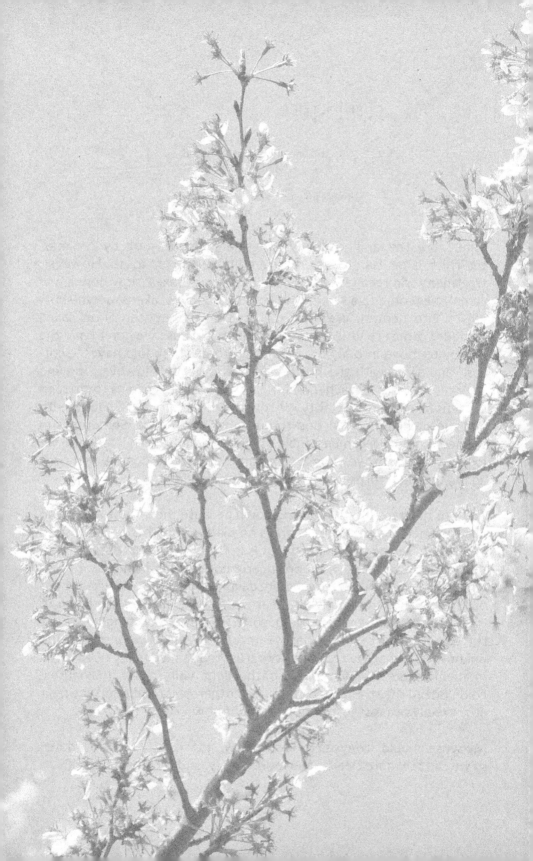

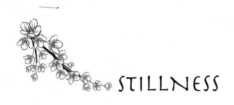 STILLNESS

Be still and know that I am God.
-Psalm 46:10

Stillness reveals the secrets of eternity.
-Lao Tzu

"Smile, breathe, and go slowly." These are simple words by Zen master Thich Nhat Hanh, yet are often difficult for us to do. However, treatment and recovery ask us to put on our brakes, slow down, and sometimes come to a screeching halt. Our body weakens, down-shifting us into neutral. We are exhausted and a new sensation called "fatigue" comes to visit. We sit in stillness because we don't have the energy to move into action and tackle "to-dos," "should haves," "got-tos," and swim with the hustle and bustle of life. However, moving slow can be a great teacher and friend. This stillness begins to sharpen our lens from a blur to clarity. We discover that born out of our breath and the silence is connection to our inner knowledge. Sometimes in stillness, the truth can become a glaring headlight in the dark and we look away. Yet, if we choose to return our gaze to it, time and time again, the glare turns into a beautiful, guiding light.

All of us need to slow everything down because there is ultimately no place we need to go. When there is no place to go, there is no rush to get anywhere and we can see what is in front of us. In the still wilderness of our treatment, we more clearly notice what brings us joy and what sinks our spirits. We feel more deeply about who and what opens our hearts and who and what creates a heavier burden. We begin to trust life to take us where we need to go instead of clinging to our rutted path. Not toward what we imagine or think we need, but the unknown of what we really do. We trust that all we really need is the moment we are in. In the middle of the night while in pain and nausea, I didn't need the strength to go to chemotherapy or radiation the next day. We always rest just right here, right now.

My sensei would always say: "Fast is slow, slow is fast." We slow down so we can see more clearly, feel more deeply, and breathe more fully.

We slow down to heal, so we are not working overtime doing everything and anything else. We slow down and settle into stillness to become more aware of who we truly are.

My journey was akin to the life of a monk on an extended retreat. Everything asked for stillness: the lack of movement needed to protect the graft, the deep healing from surgery, the rest to help the fatigue, and the calm to lessen the rising tide of nausea. I was only just eating, only just resting, only just sleeping, only just experiencing this moment of ever-changing sensations.

When we slow down, magical gifts are given to us. In stillness, I saw the individual peck of a finch at the feeder, the shift of a shadow, and the flutter of a butterfly. I sensed the lift of a robin's wings before it took flight, the rustle of an individual leaf, the footsteps of an insect, the subtle dance of the wind, and the echo of my ancestors. In stillness we connect with all things: the quiet strength of a tree, the expansiveness of an infinite blue sky, and the immovable strength of the mountain. If we are still and listen closely, we are aware of the silence of the universe and the voice of the divine. This stillness is infinite love. When we rest in stillness in both our mind and body, we discover the vast emptiness that holds us in its healing.

Time becomes meaningless in the face of stillness and illness. We exist in both one moment in time and eternity itself. This is what we want when we are on a trajectory of counting days, weeks, and months between test results, or until treatment is over. We then begin to rest, not just in the stillness of a weakened body, but the stillness and silence of a clearing mind. This stillness greets us the moment we surrender and say yes to whatever is in front of us: a doctor's appointment, an upcoming scan, or an unknown future. Stillness brings forth a thunder of inner awareness, opening the door to the infinite.

Day after day in recovery, I bowed before this sacred place of silence and stillness as my resting place. I observed but didn't act, sometimes out of choice, sometimes out of great fatigue, and often out of both. In stillness, time disappeared. In our normal frenzy and blur, we periodically come up for air and can't believe a year has ended, or it is our birthday once again. Stillness takes us to the deepest, most timeless place within, expanding us outward to eternity.

In the stillness of healing, I traveled great distances. The film of all my years rewound and I wandered through the twists and turns, back alleys, and open highways of my life. Sometimes the film unfolded freely in openness and joy and, at other times, I slammed on the emotional brakes and the film fluttered, even burned as frames jammed to a halt in the pain of remembrance. Stillness took me down deep to cavernous tunnels, where little light has shined for years. It uncovered the stings and scars, the hurts and the sorrows, along with the joy and the wonders that are held within as I go through the surface streets of my life. Stillness revealed paths that seemed perhaps not the best taken, but whose challenges led to great transformation. Stillness itself became the empty cup that embraced everything. It forgave me my sins and opened me into the vast space that holds and reveres the tiniest creature and the infinite galaxies. This is the stillness that speaks the language of silence, revealing our deepest truths for all who are brave enough to turn the volume off for the wisdom to be heard. If we can find silence and stillness during our recovery, then it will be our porthole to deeper lessons, wisdom, and inner peace. However, how many of us can dare to still both our mind and body? At times, the silence can sound thunderous and deafening.

During treatment and recovery, we are often not given a choice. We sit in stillness, too tired to move. Our bodies being forced into stillness can be frightening at first because the incessant acrobatics of our minds can be frenetic. It is one thing to be still in our bodies, but quite another to be still in our minds. Removing outside noise and distractions is much easier than removing our internal noise. In stillness, the volume heightens on our thoughts; we more clearly see all the drama that unfolds within us from moment to moment on the projection screen of our mind. What is the story being told? Is it one we truly want to watch and listen to? Would we turn to this channel of our television set? Since we have always identified more with our thoughts than our silence, this forced stillness may be our first introduction to our crazy mind and its endless high fidelity chatter. Silence allows for deep listening to the truth that is within us, but we must first remove the clamor of our thoughts. Our voice of insight and clarity is muted beneath the pinball machine of our minds and the hubbub of our lives. When we are still in both body and mind, there is no need to think. Each step reveals itself. With time, surrender, and aided with the fatigue of our journey, we begin to realize that we are not this seemingly nonstop conversation, but the stillness and beautiful gaps between the incessantly firing thoughts in our mind. If we can then open up and allow the stillness of our bodies to envelop our minds, we can be transformed by our illness.

We discover that our quiet center is always there during our recovery, no matter what we are doing or where we are. All we have to do to return to home base is to take one deep breath. This inner stillness is where we can rest during long intervals in the lobby, endless pokes from needles, and the difficult wait for the results of scans. It is with us inside the radiation tunnel, during the drip of chemotherapy, and at the center of every wave of nausea. Inhale, exhale, and we are magically there.

In this vast silence, we find ourselves. We find that we are the awareness gazing out on the movie of our lives. We are the spectators in this grand drama before us. Conditions and circumstances no longer decide how we feel. Instead we rest in the infinite veil of stillness.

In still moments, everyone and everything was here with me. All were involved in this great dance of my healing: the love of my family and friends, the blossom, the chirp of the bird, the kindness of a stranger, those still here, and those long gone. In stillness, we are all one.

We don't always understand the whys of all the unfolding events before us, but we can trust and align ourselves with life itself. In this stillness, we surrender and accept what is in front of us. We become one with what is so. We know that whatever circumstance we are in, it is there to teach us depth, compassion, knowing, and infinite trust. In the timeless stillness, we are not our illness; we can just be.

Trust the stillness. It is always there. In our humanity and untamed minds, we are often disconnected to it. Our practice is to return to it time and time again. It is always waiting patiently for us without becoming bitter and resentful. This quiet center grows old with us. It silently bears witness to our lives: the soaring take-offs and the crash landings, the soft rock of love, the cutting edge of the lie, the dangerous detours, and the safe open roads. Our quiet, still center has often lived a long life in our back alleys and basements, nowhere to be seen or felt in our lives. If we are gentle on ourselves, keep opening our heart and quieting our mind, we will find infinite grace and always be led back to it. In the wilderness of our healing, we can surround our pain, worry, and fear with this healing stillness and silent space.

Our time of recovery can actually become a time of quiet meditation where we connect not with our fears, but our deep silence and still center. It can be a time of deeper wisdom, inner peace, and intuition. Stillness becomes a best friend and a great teacher. It is always there to wrap us in its deep blanket of quiet and tranquility so we can rest in our essence and not in our illness. It is the eternal space between our worries and fears. It is the silence amid our projected thoughts of our future. We can find solace in its endless expansiveness. No matter how seemingly small the silence within the roar of pain, the cacophony of our thoughts, or the external noise of a busy hospital, let stillness be your healing anchor. As our thoughts soften and our inner stillness expands, we've come home.

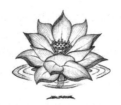

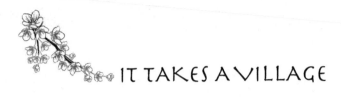

# IT TAKES A VILLAGE

Cancer affects all of us, whether you're a daughter, mother,
sister, friend, coworker, doctor, or patient.
-Jennifer Aniston

It isn't always where the road leads.
It is the love of those we meet along the way.
-Hallmark greeting card

This has not been a solo voyage. In the face of other challenges in their life events, others have been on this journey with me at the same time. It has taken a village to help me get this far and cross all the milestones. My family continued to anticipate my needs large and small, make daily drives to City of Hope despite their own hectic schedules, shop, clean, nurse, and cheer me on. All the angels of Team Suzette lovingly continued to remember me and carry me on the wings of their love, generosity, support, and constant visits through cards, letters, gifts, and contributions with each unfolding chapter of my journey. The village has truly made all the difference.

A village rises from love and is expressed in action. They arrive without expectation and with unending compassion. They are without seeming boundaries. They are family, friends, students, doctors, nurses, volunteers, acquaintances, and even those we have never met. They walk with us on our journey, step by step. The village sits with compassionate hearts at our side. They slow their pace to walk along with us. They steer our wheelchair and tenderly hold our hand. They help us wrap scarves around our bald head. When they leave us, they are still with us. They are the threads in our tapestry without which its beautiful, healing design would fall apart. They offer hope, strength, kindness, and laughter. Our village feels our pain while carrying their own aches of worry and concern. They give their gifts without fanfare and with life-changing impact.

My village carried me on their wings in both the dark of the night and the light of each passing day. The Team Suzette website was built in one day. The request for funds goal was met before I was wheeled in for surgery. The village was with me in each crackle of the radiation rays and each rise and fall of nausea. The village became my eyes, arms, and engine. They cleaned wounds and emptied my body's drains. They arranged my house, my kitchen, and my bedroom with user-friendly thoughtfulness. They shopped, chopped, and cooked. They did my wash and changed sheets. They guided me in my impaired vision. The village made their wedding plans and "to-dos" revolve around my treatment schedules. The village took plane rides from Arizona to be at my side. The village showered with me with cards and guest book messages of encouragement, generosity, love, and kindness. The village left doorstep deliveries of bouquets of flowers, a special rock, homemade organic vegetable soup, endless avocados, and loving gifts. The village placed pillows gingerly under my arms, walked with me along the seashore, washed each dish, put eye drops lovingly and carefully in my paralyzed eye, and tossed prayers upward for deep healing and miracles. The village filled my backyard with cheer and love. They carried me to the healing stillness of Cambria with their compassion as my engine. The village took me to the end of the pier at the finish of radiation and chemotherapy to watch the sun and the end of my treatments sink into the horizon. The love of my village continued to open me to deeper and deeper healing. The village of doctors, nurses, and support staff propelled me throughout my surgery and my treatment with great care, expertise, and tenderness. The village made my life more peaceful and surrounded by grace so I could heal more deeply. My village still carries me on the wings of their love with each unfolding chapter, varying needs for encouragement, support, and adapting to ever-changing sensations and realities.

I used to think of myself as independent. I've been self-employed without anyone's safety net beneath me for most of my life. I've traveled on solo adventures overseas. I've packed up my art and displays and driven countless miles alone to exhibit in fine art shows throughout the United States. I've sculpted my life from the depths of my passion and desire to live from my heart and soul. However, if any of us think we are independent, we are living a false reality that can be directly shattered at any moment by illness or circumstance.

It may not be easy to embrace the village at first, as it asks us to let go and surrender. If we have lived a life of seeming independence, it may be difficult to accept help, generosity, or even deep and abiding love. Yet the realities of recovery often give us no choice. In the free fall of diagnosis and treatment, we are asked to let go and surrender to our village. I needed help. I could not have taken one step of this journey by myself. The Affordable Care Act, the skill of the doctors, compassionate hands of the nurses, the loving care of the medical therapists, and Team Suzette family and friends reaching out to each and every need, all carried me on the wings of their love. My village was with me moment to moment. I had an arm in a sling, a patch on my eye, and a precariously healing graft. I was unable to cook, shop, drive and walk any distance alone. I could cling to wanting to be independent, or I could let go in gratitude and love to all the ways everyone was there for me.

If we accept what is and let go of our way of doing things, we can open to all the endless acts of kindness with great appreciation and reverence. If we can embrace our dependency, we learn deep lessons in how to freely accept what is given, how to state what we need, how to bow in deep humility, and how we have truly never been independent. Each strand in our village is needed, whether it is within the immediate village that surrounds us during our recovery, or the vastness of the infinite village.

It takes a village to go through treatment. It takes a village to go through life. It is not six degrees of separation. Separation is an illusion. Now I look around me and see my reliance and my dependence on everything and everyone. We stand on the shoulders of our ancestors. I was never independent. The beat of my heart has always been connected to the pulse of all who have come before me. None of us are a solo act. The props on the stage of life are built by the hands of many. Each step we take throughout the day is from the grace of the village. I look at the world now and I see all the intricate and interconnected threads that make up my life.

We may isolate and claim independence, but each life is a twinkling star that couldn't exist without every other star in the constellation. The village is a tsunami crashing over me in its magnitude, its wonder, its breath-taking gifts, and its inspiring spirit. It is an eternity of people, places, and things that cradle me with great love. I look at my sisters and I see the love of our parents and my parents' parents, going forever backward in time. I bow to each sacrifice, each lesson given, all their blood, sweat, and tears, their triumphs and losses, and all the love that still shines from them from beyond the veil. When I see my doctors, I see the gifts given from their parents, every teacher along their path, the authors of each book they read, and all their discipline and passion. I turn on a light. I no longer see just an illuminated bulb, but every strand in the village that brought this gift to me. I may have the independence of purchasing food and cooking a meal, but I am nothing without the farmer, the truck driver, the packer, the picker, or the store and its employees. I came into this world not only through the love of my mother and father, but through the skill of the doctor who delivered me, those who built the hospital, and the nurses who assisted me down the birth canal. The list is endless.

Life in its great wisdom and mystery has somehow designed the circumstances and challenges of being here to require us to need each other. I have endless gratitude to my village for their constant love, ever-abiding light, prayers, and selfless generosity. I rest in immense appreciation for the vast village of existence. I tip my heart and soul in infinite thanks to my eternal village beyond the veil. As we travel throughout our journey, let us remember that we are a part of everyone's village as they are also a part of ours. Let us see the faces of each other as our face, reach out our hands to another as they reach out to us, and continue to give thanks to all, knowing we are all in this healing village together.

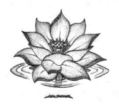

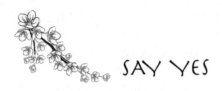 SAY YES

And the day came when the risk to remain tight in a bud
was more painful than the risk it took to blossom.
-Anaïs Nin

Whatever comes, accept it. Whatever goes, accept it.
-Sri Swami Satchidananda

How do we stay open and say "yes" amid the sting, the fear, the slamming door, and the closed fist of the "no" in the cancer journey? How do we fling our hearts open in the midst of pain, weakness, and sometimes despair? How do we stay open to a frightening diagnosis, the ever-excruciating wait for test results, going fifteen rounds in the ring with chemotherapy, the deep insult of surgery, the radioactive glucose injected with each PET scan, scarves around bald heads, the crackle of radiation in a dark tunnel, and the unfolding great unknown of our journey?

Cancer is yet another circumstance of our lives. We are all continually surrounded by the unfolding of both pain and wonder in our journeys. We are caught between the slam of our brakes and the push of our accelerator. Opening. Closing. Sometimes we don't want to say either yes or no. Instead, we want to turn down a darkened alley to avoid all reality. We may speed through, slow to a stop, or detour to evade what is in front of us, but in the jack-in-the-box of our lives all will eventually and often unexpectedly rise to the surface once again.

That our hearts will open and close during the often chaotic ride of our lives isn't to be denied. However, every moment is our opportunity to swing the door open once again and reconnect to ourselves, to others, and to this world by choosing to say yes.

Saying yes means accepting the unacceptable. We do not have to like what we see or feel, but we accept it as what is so in each precious moment of our lives. Victor Frankl remains the champion of saying yes. During his imprisonment, he made each moment count. When he was released, the depths of his compassion rippled outward to humanity in both his actions and his written words.

We must embrace our circumstances and bring meaning to each moment. These are hard words to swallow, but it is not our circumstances that create most of our pain and suffering, but our mind wanting things to be another way. Our journey of healing is a great schoolhouse to learn how to say yes. Diagnosis and recovery challenge us to remain open and to accept the reality before us.

It takes courage to say yes and look at our life circumstances face-to-face and eye-to-eye. However, if we close the curtain, there is darkness. How can we then see, experience, and learn from what is in front of us? We need to keep getting up, keep opening up, and keep saying yes, even though we initially scream no. Circumstances remain; they come and go. If we were fearful, resisted, and said no every time, we would have never ventured down the dark, foreboding, and bumpy birth canal into the light of our lives.

Saying yes means staying open to every up and down, seeming insult, challenge, and twist and turn. Embracing any journey, however difficult, can make a heavy heart light and a difficult road smoother. In saying yes, we let go of negativity and resistance. If we are in the moment, not judging, not resisting, and accepting what is, then we intuitively know what to do. We accept what is happening and let this surrender absorb all into its timeless, infinite, and loving heart.

In order to feel the pleasure, we have to also feel the pain. To be open and not resist our discomfort means that we can also be open to joy and wonder. We can't pick and choose what to be open to: We need to experience all of life. If not, the result is our suffering. Saying no closes the door to love and miracles.

When my face and neck looked like an old tree bark, brittle and chipped, I said, "Yes, this is just what is so right now," and tiny spaces of smoothness were revealed.

When swallowing was difficult, I said "yes" and it softened the edges of the food making its way down my throat.

When my throat was sore, mouth parched as a desert wind, and taste metallic and foreign from radiation, I said yes, letting it be my experience for that moment in time.

When the tissue hardened tighter and tighter and severed muscles and nerves restricted my mouth from barely opening, I said yes and thank you to the small opening that still welcomed food.

As my sister guided me with my blurred vision and rising tides of nausea to the elevator leading to the radiation department, saying yes opened me and let her words of inspiration and love embrace me.

As I gingerly put scissors in my hand to try and cut my art materials after just removing my sling, I said yes and gave great gratitude for a single splice.

When I was waiting in the lobby for hours, I said yes and time disappeared.

While sitting in limited motion in my backyard and wanting to move with wild abandon, I said yes and took flight with the birds.

When struggling hard to put a sweatshirt over my head, I relaxed, said yes, and it slid more easily onto my body.

When my mind did its wild dance of thinking about past and future, saying yes let me rest in emptiness, stillness, and the present moment.

When my body and mind wanted to shut out the pain and anxiety, saying yes allowed me to open up and feel all the love, kindness, and compassion given to me throughout my healing journey.

When saying yes, I could lie on the conveyor belt and actually experience the beauty of the lit ceiling panel of cherry blossoms. Saying yes relaxed and opened me while the infusions of chemotherapy slowly seeped into my body.

Saying yes allowed me to enter the doors of City of Hope, sensing the valiant energy of the patients and the love of the many volunteers, many of whom had been through their own struggles and triumphed.

Saying yes brought light, space, and comfort into the dark of my night. Electrifying sensations exploding, nerves seemingly trapped in tiny dead-end streets, and muscles jammed together like bumper cars with no place to go, all softened inside the yes. When I said "yes," the fireworks inside me would become a single, solitary shooting comet blazing across an expansive night sky.

Saying yes emptied me to the infinity that holds all the stars, like a million eyes, blinking at me from above. By saying yes, I became the vast endless sky.

During our treatment, we are often pushed beyond our limits. Our body wants to rest and stare at a tree. Saying yes offers us the space to relax and heal. By saying yes, we honor our body and let it lead us to what is best for our recovery. We trust in the unfolding, step-by-step, and breath-by-breath.

No matter how tired, despairing, or weak, we need to keep opening up, time and time again. We need to keep softening instead of hardening. We must continue to remove our armor, since it doesn't really protect us. Instead, it keeps us from feeling and experiencing life. Saying yes is to be open to healing.

Saying yes does not mean you don't say no first. To truly say yes, it means we have first known the underbelly of no. We have learned how to look at the no squarely in the face. Know thy enemy, know thyself. Yes is born from no. How do we know courage if we haven't faced the fear that arises in the dark of the night? We can't know hope if we haven't tasted despair, acceptance if we haven't wrestled with denial, and peace if we haven't ignited in anger and rage. To know the positive light, we must have come face to face with the sting of negativity and the black hole of darkness. Clarity is born of confusion. Strength and resiliency come from falling and rising again and again. From loneliness we discover we are all one. This is our healing journey. This is our spiritual journey.

Saying yes is to surrender to whatever falls in our paths. Saying yes is moving with grace, gratitude, and trusting that all is for our greatest good. We trust that what lies before us is our path to discovering deeper meaning and purpose. We realize that healing is a many layered journey, and that a "cure" can be a very blessed and joyous but narrow box. True healing is the depth, width, and breadth that we open our hearts, quiet our wild minds, embrace our true spirits, and experience our deep connection with each other. We are then cured of our tiny self, our narrow views, and petty clinging. Healing is trusting, letting go, and surrendering to this moment and to all that never changes. In saying a resounding *yes* we realize that to live or to die is not the question or the most important outcome. Instead, it is the grace and freedom we are given as we rise up and experience the gift of each precious moment.

We all come with our baggage, scripts, and emotional reflexes that we have gathered, cherished, and protected over the years. We can all think back to situations that used to anger us, but now the fuse has lengthened or even disappeared altogether. Saying yes means separating what is a kernel of true emotion from our attachment to the soap opera of our circumstances. We all fall victim to this. Saying yes allows us to leave the drama behind so we can stay connected to what is true right here and right now. We rest in our awareness of, not our identity with, the changing emotional tide of our lives.

Once we come to know how to center and ground ourselves, we can more easily face our challenges with a yes. We begin to learn our lessons, let go, soften, and go beyond. We are not unlike children who fall off of their bicycles, then learn to slow down over a big bump. We mount once more to feel the breeze on our face, our legs move like pistons propelling us forward, and our spirits soar. What our parents said or didn't say loses its grip. What someone does or doesn't do is drained of its power. When life doesn't go our way, we follow its current instead. We say yes and no longer feel like a toy boat tossed around in the turbulent emotional sea of our lives. The ever-unfolding dramatic antics of our minds that demand to be on center stage begin to soften and even disappear. We recognize their foreplay and we don't engage. We see how saying no closes the shutters and moves us away from the light. When we shine the light of "yes," the "no" of our false nature is uncovered and shattered with illumination. We begin to watch the antics of our minds as if they are passing storm clouds that no longer gather momentum from our fears and worries. We calmly say, "Oh, there you are again. There you go." We begin to trust that the sky is always blue behind the clouds of our passing thoughts. We become the sky. With time, we have more and more space for forgiveness, for letting go, and for saying yes.

If we stick around on this planet long enough, we have endless opportunities to learn. Our healing journey is our master teacher. If we can become the observer to the melodrama of our illness, whether through meditation, prayer, therapy, or resting in stillness, we begin the work of taming the frenzy in our minds. We are human; saying no can continue to call to us, but we don't give it a power and permanence. Circumstances come to visit, but we greet them all with acceptance and letting go. We don't become bitterness, fear, or resentment. We no longer get snarled in the undertow. We learn to stay on the surface and swim across the emotional current without being dragged out to sea.

In time we become snake charmers to our writhing and hissing mind. When we open beyond its antics, we can then embrace both the weed and the flower, each with their lesson, each with their gift. We do not have to deny anything. We understand deeply, we forgive, we learn, and we are able to let go and say yes.

Growing up in an alcoholic family, I lived with the trauma of emotional land mines exploding unexpectedly. I developed a raw antenna to detect any nuances in the shifts of energy at home. I learned how to contract and armor myself at a moment's notice, in order to shield me from all the unpredictable outbursts surrounding me. We train our muscles well to seemingly protect us from feeling what is in front of us, to say no to both emotional and physical pain. However, the resistance just hardens us and we never fully feel both deep pain and great pleasure.

We all have this knee-jerk emotional reaction to different things in our lives. We all wear our armor. It's understandable. Treatment, scans, and constant follow-ups challenge our ability to say yes. Simply moving through each day with its small emotional insults and stresses can contract our minds and muscles. We need to have a practice that continues to remind our body and our hearts to open. For me, twenty years of tai chi, meditation, energy work, connection with nature, reflection, and prayer have been my paths in continuing to open my mind, body, and spirit and say yes to life, time and time again. The important thing is just continuing to open. Our practice is to keep moving past the fear, the seeming injustice, and the pain and say yes to whatever is happening. We must remember, until we no longer forget, to keep our heart open so healing light and love can continue to move through us.

It is work to keep opening up time and time again. The heart will open and close. We must not deny the no, but we need to keep reminding ourselves that every moment is an opportunity to reconnect with life and love. Saying yes allows us to rewind and reflect and find a way to open to even the worst sting, insult, and discomfort. We realize that instead of protecting us from pain, the no makes our suffering worse while the yes will always soften us into deeper peace and healing.

Our journey of diagnosis and treatment is a challenging practice. Saying yes doesn't mean we have to like our diagnosis, our treatment, and the curve ball of our circumstances. It does mean that we continue to accept what is happening at just this moment. We open to the pierce of the IV needle, a wave of nausea, a fear in the dark of the night, along with the gentle hug of a loved one, words of encouragement, and the rising sun. At the end of each day, we must ask ourselves: "Where and when did I close down? How can I open again and say yes instead of no?" Always we must seek to open wider and wider to everyone and everything; family and friends, the tiny goldfinch, the ever expansive sky, and all the mystery beyond the veil.

Saying no will not change the drip of chemotherapy, the rays of radiation, or the result of our scans. It will tighten and contract us and make us feel small. We throw our energy away with worry and most of our projections are scenarios we create that never come true. When we say yes, there is no friction added to our challenges. We no longer fall into the dramatic antics of our mind but become the vast awareness watching the movie of our lives with a still and quiet center.

Saying yes allowed me to open up to feel my best friend, Chuck, whom I longed to be here for the journey, beside me as a soft place to fall in the deep of the night. I felt the unconditional love of my sweet angel Tattoo surrounding me with her peace. I could feel the energy of the universe and the infinite pulsating through me. I could feel the deep compassion of all of the Team Suzette family and friends carrying me on the wings of their love. Saying yes allowed me to move from form to spirit and receive love and light. Saying yes reminded me to return to the breath, time and time again. Saying yes opened me to miracles of healing.

Saying yes is continually reminding ourselves that we are on a magnificent and mysterious journey that is life. Saying yes is to be present in our lives with a grateful heart. We accept what comes, but also accept what goes. Our work is to keep loving ourselves and love being here, no matter what is put in our path. All our resistance, our craziness, our illness, and our fears then become our greatest teachers.

We are here to add whatever love we can muster into the mix. If we do not recoil in fear, indifference, or pain, then each day in our lives is made up of connection, compassion, and openness to everything and everyone. If we continue to say yes to even the smallest opening and follow the light, even if imagined, we will find our freedom. Then we continue to say yes, because we now know that nothing, not pain, not illness, and not fear, can touch our spirit. This is expressed in the inspiring poem "Cancer is so Limited."

It cannot cripple love.
It cannot shatter hope.
It cannot corrode faith.
It cannot eat away peace.
It cannot destroy confidence.

It cannot kill friendship.
It cannot shut out memories.
It cannot silence courage.
It cannot invade the soul.
It cannot reduce eternal life.
It cannot quench the spirit.
It cannot cancel resurrection.

-Robert L. Lynn

When we can reach a place where we say yes genuinely and complete-ly, and bow to each life situation as our teacher without a label of good or bad, we are resilient warriors and masters of our own being.

By saying yes, we keep moving beyond the slap, the sting, the punch, and the contraction. Time and time again. Eventually letting go and opening up becomes our natural way. Everything becomes both a gift and a lesson. Saying yes is our freedom.

We must become like Frankl and his fellow prisoners, reaching out to share their last cherished crumbs of bread with one another. We must say yes to our challenges. They are endless. They are our freedom. They are our healing.

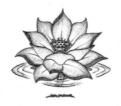

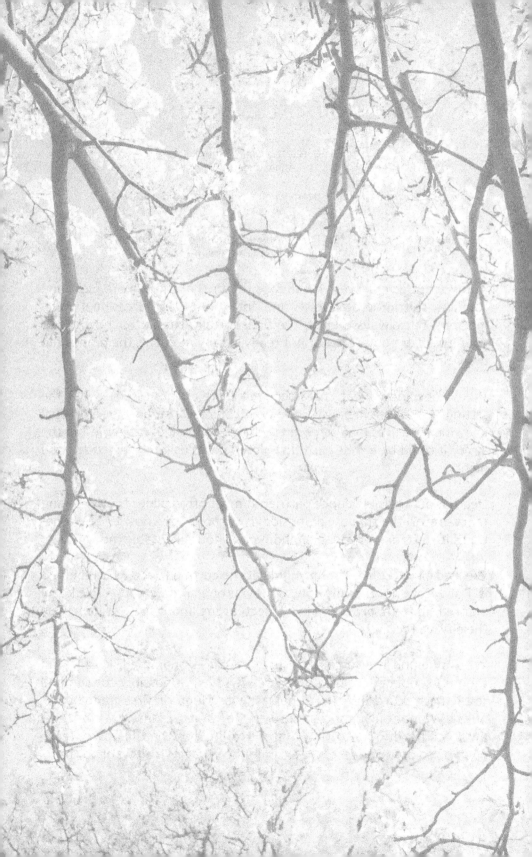

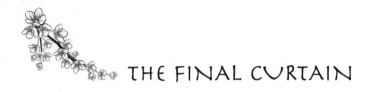

# THE FINAL CURTAIN

Death is just birth in disguise.
-Annie Kagan

How can we know death when we don't know how to live?
-Confucious

Eternity is not something that begins after you are dead. It is going on all the time.
-Charlotte Perkins Gilman

In the script of our lives, we all face the final act. There are plots and conflicts, shifting protagonists and antagonists, and occasional inter-missions, but always there is the final curtain. No matter how old or young, rich or poor, ready or not ready, at any moment, the drapes can draw closed.

We do not know what characters will share our last scene, what the setting will be, or when it is coming. It could be a surprise or a gradual knowing. Our lives may screech to a halt, the smell of rubber left in the air, or it could be a wide turn that slowly eases us into the gentle good night.

Death is our invisible dance partner. It most often glides footloose and fancy-free in the shadow alongside us without our knowledge. Some-times it steps on our toes, reminding us of our inevitable mortality.

We lead our lives like Toto, tugging at the curtain to see who is behind it. But we are never really able to draw it open for a glimpse. We kneel before it in faith, proclaim and reflect, argue and insist, yet never see the elusive face.

Who is behind the curtain? Jesus, Buddha, Mohammad, Krishna, all the saints, nobody, or nothing? Are we saved or possibly condemned to the flesh-scorching fires of hell as I was taught in first grade by the nuns? We not only want an answer, we want *the* answer. If not, we must fall headfirst into the mystery of life and the unknown. If we open up to only one face, we exclude the other. We all want to call what happens after the final curtain by name. In our humanity, we want to define, categorize, and separate. We want to be right.

We move through life as if we are given a guarantee. Yet, on the package and in the small print, it clearly states that we can self-destruct at any time. There is no planned obsolescence, no predictable last breath. We all have the period at the end of the sentence, no matter how rambling and long.

Death is the image we see on the television screen. It flickers on and off of our radar, mostly off. Death happens to a parent, sometimes even a spouse or friend. Not us. If we see it out of the corner of our eyes, we quickly glance in the opposite direction. We only see what we look at and we don't make eye contact with death. Then one day, we suffer emotional whiplash when it comes to visit.

If we are honest, anyone who has had a diagnosis of cancer or gone on the journey with a loved one, or perhaps anyone who just hears the word cancer, has the letters "D-E-A-T-H" slide across their consciousness. Images flash on the slide projection screen of our mind; bald heads, IV drips, hospices, and the final amen. When the diagnosis comes, it is hard to escape the fact that death now rides shotgun with us. It is sometimes a silent passenger and then, quite suddenly, it can also start to give us directions like an unwanted backseat driver.

Illness awakens us from a seeming lifetime slumber to face our own mortality. We look around and ask ourselves, "Who am I? How did I get here? Where do I go from here?" How we face our eventual death is our greatest lesson if we choose to continue learning. How do we say *yes* to what can feel like the ultimate *no*? The face of death begins to move us from form to spirit, from the familiar to the unknown. Perhaps the more we have clung to the familiar, the more difficult it is to stare at the ultimate unknown face-to-face. How do we ever gracefully let go of this body that has defined us, expressed us, and has seemingly been us for a lifetime?

My dance with the face of death has greatly changed its footwork over my lifetime. The first dead person I saw was at age seven, a great aunt who died of a heart attack. The motion picture in my mind rolls the film backward and the reel flickers at the image of a child with deep wandering eyes, paisley skirt, navy blue sweater, shiny patent leather shoes with gold buckles, a black prayer cap, and deep confusion in her heart. She faints when she sees her great aunt's opaque, stiff body in the coffin. My childish mind and heart hears bits and pieces of adult conversations about her last moments as she was unable to reach the phone to call for help and died alone. The words echo off the mortuary walls and bounce around in my mind like a pinball. Where is her hearty laugh, her earthy smell, and her wide eyes?

When I was fifteen, my grandma died. After her funeral, it was as if death had somehow escaped from the coffin, at the moment of her burial before the final prayer. It was with me in the car as my parents drove home, sat with me at the dining room table, and woke me in the deep of the night. I would open my eyes and see its blackness and then knew why people were afraid of the dark. I would wonder if death had followed the others home as well. Did it sneak into their purses, ride home in their ashtrays, or slip into their trunks as an unknowing passenger? Did it enter their front doors as an unexpected and uninvited guest? Did it leave them the moment they put their black slacks and dresses on hangers and turned on their favorite TV programs? For me, it was the guard on watchful duty twenty-four hours a day. Just when I thought it was gone, I would see it staring back at me out of the mashed potatoes on my dinner plate.

How do I say what it was like? I couldn't give death a voice. It seemed to have reached its bony hand into my throat and pulled out my vocal chords. I didn't know its language. How could I describe it? And most of all, who (if anyone) could I tell about this monster?

It was an obsessive boyfriend, following my every move, calling uninvited, tucking itself under my sheets each night.

In the bathroom, it glistened in the vein-splicing edge of the razor blades. It taunted me in the childproof cap of the aspirin bottle, which beckoned me to swallow them, joining hand-in-hand with death.

It was in the blood red on the Mercurochrome bottle, the poison sign of the drain cleaner, and in an easy slip in the bathtub.

It sat on my night stand, shining out from the florescent hands of the ticking clock. It lured me with its bait of permanent stillness, a final escape, no more questions, ultimate answers, and a time-out. I tried to corral it, define it, and break its spirit like a wild horse. I looked for a stronger voice than mine to tame it. I went to church but it reminded me of a funeral.

In school, the teachers taught death. In English literature, we read T. S. Eliot's "The Hollow Men": "In this valley of dying stars / In this hollow valley / This broken jaw of our lost kingdoms." In science class we dissected dead frogs. During Spanish class we subjugated the verb "to die"—yo mori, tu moriste, ella murio, nosotros morimos, and ellan murieron. In PE class, I tried to exercise, but my limbs were dying and one of my feet was in the grave. Death stepped out from the vertical hold of the television set and joined me for dinner. It had a leash around my neck and took me for a walk after the evening meal.

I wondered. What if death was a grand facade and not the doorway to a permanent refuge? What if it was really a porthole leading to all the pain we tried to evade in life? What if it was a mirror that reflected back to us each numbed hurt, each unkind thought, and each action stopped by the brake pedal of fear? The atheists saw death as "dead, buried, and on the third day, the flowers wilted." The religious saw it as the resurrection. What if it was neither the final respite nor the final act, but the final truth within ourselves?

I had become so fearful and consumed with death that I had never truly stopped to stare life squarely in the face. Surely there was the flip side, even though it felt like death was a two-headed coin in the toss. The power of death came from its ultimate mystery and its ultimate power to take away everything in an instant. However, the trump card that life had on its side was being right here, right now. So I took off death's black mask and met it eye-to-eye, face-to-face. I began to discover the pulse of life.

What did it enjoy for dinner? What were its moods, needs, and joys? What did it require for survival? By defining it, I began to define myself. Life began to beckon me every time I reached out with an open hand and heart. It began to tuck me into the warm embrace of my soft sheets and blanket each night, did cartwheels with me on the lawn, and reveled in my laughter. My joy brought joy to life. My dreams were the hopes and dreams of life itself. I looked in the mirror and saw life. It said hello with each wink of my eye, curl of my hair, flush in my cheeks, and smile on my lips. It was in the power of my legs pedaling my bike throughout the neighborhood, the belly laugh that turned to tears in the company of friends, and the smell of homemade chocolate chip cookies. When I sang, life sang through me. I began to see the face of life superimposed on the face of death. They seemed somehow woven together on the same tapestry. Finally, I saw not only the thorn and wilted flower, but the eternal return of the magnificent rose. Life and I had become one and the same. I found the power of choice. I said yes to life.

Perhaps our diagnosis makes us the chosen ones who are allowed to go on this healing journey. Our illness rouses us from our slumber, awakening to the precious gift of our lives. We look at death eye-to-eye, so we must also look at our lives face-to-face. We no longer move through our days in a hypnotic dream. Who else is given three and six month reprieves on their lives and a prognosis for survival? Who else has percentages attributed to their possible time on this planet, with words like "terminal" and "survivor" as brands on their chest? "We lost him to cancer"; what other disease is most likely to define itself after speaking of a loved one's death? Who else sees such fear in the stunned eyes of each person with whom they share their diagnosis? Who else must then listen to the long list of all those the person has lost to the same illness? Who else faces, in one solitary breath of diagnosis, a head-on collision with just this precious moment in time?

How many of us have gone to the cliff's edge and looked into the seemingly black abyss of death? What few have resided in that place where death looms, not as a distant blur, but magnified, allowing one to notice the intricacies and magnificence of every rock, weed, and flower as if for the first time? During my recovery, I have faced the final curtain where the aperture closes to a tiny opening, yet also widens to empty into eternity. If we can find peace and acceptance in the final curtain, we can say yes to death and an even more thunderous yes to life.

In facing the final curtain, it is easy to feel cheated of a guarantee we never had. Our diagnosis and prognosis catapults us into the foreboding possibility of death. However, that also makes us face what is real and true as well as what is temporary in our lives. Death is indeed our greatest teacher and illuminating reality. It can snatch away everything that we once thought we were: our possessions, our roles, our triumphs, and our seemingly precious identities. In one breath, all disappears. Death is the grand checkout counter as we seem to leave everything behind. Or do we?

What does death ask of us? Simply, it asks us to live before we die. Shouldn't we be thankful to the final curtain for its grand wake-up call?

On this journey, I now travel closer to the edge. Questions of life and death raise their hands like eager students wanting to be acknowledged. What is this life of ours? Does it have a pulse all its own or do we create the rhythm? Are we the unwilling dance partner, forever stepping on its feet because we haven't learned our lessons, or slowed down enough to embrace the melody and hear the tune? Do we reach out to take its hand and expect it to lead, then complain when we can't follow its footsteps? Can we not even hear the music and recognize the beat in the clutter and clamor of our life? And who ever really gets up to dance?

What is this gift of life wrapped in a mysterious paper, bow, and ribbon, which holds both the dark night of the soul and divine light of love? Inside is the hand of the beggar, the steady stare of the catatonic, the wounded body, the sting of the lie, the slap on the face, the leap that falls short, the bloated belly of the starving child, and death by loneliness. Yet, within the box is also the innocent child, the laughter, the smooth rock of love, the wedding vow, the clasped hands of the lover, the sweet smile, and the rise of the morning sun. Each experience is a gift given, but how many of us choose to unwrap it?

Where do I fit within this box in the fleeting moment that is my life? My box is my humanity, which is a miraculous gift. I am also a spiritual being in this human garment seeking to be more and more an instrument of the divine. Birth and death are only portholes and not fixed points in time. I hold the hand of the hospice patient on one side and newborn child on the other. Each of them seems to give the other their existence and I am but the pulse of both. Out of the mud of my humanity grows the divine lotus blossom.

Where is my dad, whom I lost to cancer? Does his spirit settle in the warm embers of my heart? Does it blow like the wind, wrapping its arms around me in a loving embrace? Does it connect with the skewed telescope of my own vision? Does he visit as a passing feeling of his nearness as I go about the ins and outs of life? Does he reside in an old photograph, the comfort of his tattered green Ireland sweater I wear, the racing form, and the genius of his beloved Whitman? Does he inhabit all of those whose lives he touched? Does his spirit fly in the heavens and see and feel my hopes, dreams, sorrows, and fears as I stumble like an infant, taking baby steps on earth as I grope my way toward eternity? Does he reside in the period, the question mark, or the et cetera? Does his spirit linger with me on the melancholic notes of the saxophone that plays to my soul?

Does he exist in a place that sees, hears, and feels beyond anything that I can fathom in my very limited humanity? Is he there in the silence of my recovery that strips away all outside distractions? Does his spirit live forever etched in my memories? I remember him in front of our house gardening and chatting with neighbors, his delight in making little cracker sandwiches of cheese and mayo in the kitchen, and him sitting in his sofa chair, reading his beloved books and studying the racing form. I remember the small but treasured gifts of a few dollars or some candy and gum that he would slip into my hand, as an adult, each time that I drove home and him patiently waiting to go inside until I was completely out of his view. I remember his smile, his laugh, and his wry humor that would rise to all occasions. I remember him playing ball with his beloved dog in the backyard and also rushing out to help my mother carry in the groceries at the first sound of her car in the driveway. I remember the stories of his life teaching in his class-room and his guiding me in how to best express myself through the written word. I remember his kindness and sensitivity as he reached out to touch the hands of all who sat in the halls of the nursing home when we visited my grandmother. In these memories and our love, he lives forever.

The most important question seems to be: How do we say yes to death, both ours and those we love? How do we embrace such ultimate uncertainty and insecurity? If we have always pushed away the unknown, it creates an even deeper crevasse, a larger leap to the other side. One of the Arabic words for "human" means "one who forgets." Yet accepting death is our ultimate freedom. No matter what our beliefs, or the state of our current health, we need to make friends with the face behind the curtain. Better now than at the final hour as the drapes draw to a close.

If life is truly about learning to say yes to what we are given, time and time again, then we have to say yes to not only life, but death itself. Then we are truly free to stare cancer or any challenge, including our own death, in the face without fear or hesitation. To live well is to die well. We need to say yes to the final curtain.

Whatever our faith or lack thereof, death can be our ally to remind us to deeply love, always learn, say what needs to be said, and do what needs to be done. It beckons us to listen more closely, breathe more deeply, and embrace life more fully. It is our master teacher, teaching us to live each day as if it was our last.

How do we prepare for death? Saying yes to death means realizing that, ultimately, we will lose it all. We prepare for death by letting go of what we think we need and who we think we are. We "die a thousand deaths." We die to our fears, pride, anger, resistance, resentments, pettiness, and desires. We surrender our insignificant clingings, the clamor in our minds, our little personalities, and connect more fully to the spirit within us, which can never die. We practice dying every day and keep opening up to what can never die. Time and time again. Saying yes to death means realizing we are not who we thought we were.

Our inner light shines brighter and brighter as we continue to let go. Then the light that was always there, blocked by the antics of our mind, is free to illuminate our entire being. We come home, but not as we have been trained to think during the final moments as we pass into the gentle good night. Instead we realize that we have always been home. We can then see from the eye of the soul as our minds drop deeply into our hearts. If we die before we die, we can live more fully in the embracing of each moment. We find heaven on earth. Our spirit is then free to soar with the divine, right here, right now.

When my dad died, flip sides of the same coin were momentarily both facing outward. At the moment of his death, I felt him hugging not only his long-gone father and mother, but also his brothers lost to war, tuberculosis, and polio. Simultaneously, I felt the huge tidal wave of unbearable sorrow in the tears of my mother, my sisters, and myself. We wanted to keep holding my dad's still warm hand, touching his forehead, talking to him, and freezing time. Beyond the veil, others longed to embrace and welcome him. In that moment, there was no separation between life and death. The shadow and the light joined in one beautiful circle of eternity. Deep heartache and seeming finality blended with joy and reunion. The good-bye was also a homecoming.

We know not our final hour, whether it be in pain, peace, chaos, or connected to our own still center. What is most important is that we face it without judgment and with abiding love. There is no perfect death. Our death will be our own individual ending to our play.

Behind the final curtain is the eternal heartbeat of everyone. It is the beat of the open heart, joining us with the beat and the symphony of the divine. Love is the universal melody for all of us. We are all one in an open and radiant heart. Eternal love is behind the final curtain, but also in front of it: the love of Jesus, the love of Buddha, the love of Mohammad, the love of those gone before, and the love of all those who remain.

The final act is the curtain call to follow our hearts home. It is the welcome mat on an open door of giving and receiving love in an endless revolving circle.

In the final act, all boundaries disappear. The garment of our body fades like a tattered, thinning, and well-worn shirt, and our divine light shines through brighter and brighter. This is the same light that beams underneath all our garments. Saying yes to death, now or at the moment of our departure, is saying yes to life.

We never stop being alive, form and spirit. We are on our journey as humans always seeking to ignite sparks of the divine within us. We are all only toddlers here learning how to walk. During our journey we rise, stumble, fall, and seek to rise again and again. In the final act, we no longer get up, but rise into the eternity of now.

Love is greater than death.

The final curtain is really the opening act.

The journey is everything—and the journey never ends.

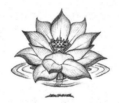

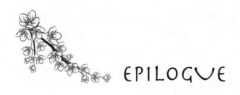# EPILOGUE

Some ask: "What will you do now? Art? Writing? Teaching?" While all have been pondered and some have returned, ultimately it no longer truly matters. It is not the details but the broader brush strokes of my life that I seek. I long to feel my life as an abstract painting with sweeps of color, movement, and texture that express:

> a return of the love given to me,
> a connection with everyone and everything,
> a deeper and deeper friendship with nature,
> a soul free to breathe, expand, and shine,
> an embrace of the gift of each day without looking to the next,
> a heart opening wider and wider as my compass to truth north,
> and a deeper experience of the divine.

What will I do now? What shall we all do? Perhaps no matter for any of us. In the words of the great author Walt Whitman: "Do anything, but let it produce joy."

Here is to opening our hearts, connecting as one, and dancing in joy! The journey is everything: five months, five years, or fifty years. What is important is right in front of us.

We can all become instruments of divine love, healing, peace, and light in whatever our circumstances. We need only say yes and be open to what is given to us. Then miracles are free to be received in grace and gratitude.

I am a work in progress: opening, closing, holding on, and letting go. This book is my compass to true north. Sometimes I am here, my feet on the ground. Other times I am caught in the riptide of life. More and more, I have learned how to float and not resist. I can bow to the day and feel its stillness and expansiveness, take what is given to me with out judgment but in thanks, trust the 360° panorama of the divine, and connect heart-to-heart with the world.

On my deathbed, I am not going to remember the difficulty of the buckle and bolt of the radiation mask, the waves of nausea from chemotherapy, the insult of surgery, or the pain in the dark of the night. I will remember my sister's words of "having my back," gentle driving over the bumps, hand clasps and I love you's, thoughtful gifts from the heart received in joy, outpourings of generosity as my safety net, and ever-so-welcomed doorstep deliveries. I will remember the ways Team Suzette family and friends carried me on the wings of their love, their simple yet profound words of encouragement, a homemade bowl of soup made from the heart, a tender touch on a weakened body, all the small but huge acts of kindness, and each miracle given to me in infinite grace and love.

I don't need to know anything. I have no need to be this or that. How do I then make a difference with my gift of life? Maybe I just become more and more of who I truly am and expand out to all with love, compassion, presence, and an open heart. Is that enough? More and more I think yes; that is actually all there is.

Unfolding twists and turns await me if I am open to them. I must listen. Be still. Reflect. Open. Embrace.

I know not how many more moments in time I will be given. I do know that I want to make every moment count, and healing is measured not in the number of our days, but by the expanse of our heart.

I light a candle now. It flickers and illuminates peace as my heart widens to embrace everyone: the prisoner in solitary confinement, the homeless person holding a request for help, the dying, and the just born. A tear of joy and gratitude slowly makes its way down my cheek as I feel every expression of encouragement, each prayer, each baby step involved in each leap forward, each kind guest book message, and each positive thought. I feel the heart of each person who graced me with their love, generosity, and support throughout my healing path and of each of you who have taken the time to read these words.

Let us all embrace and cherish this gift of life. Whatever our circumstances, whatever our paths. Let us give meaning to whatever is in front of us and allow it to remind us to open our heart, connect more deeply, expand our senses, vibrate with beauty and laughter, embrace the mystery, appreciate the journey, and find heaven on earth.

I wrote this prayer in my journal after my diagnosis:

> May this journey free me to become a better person, lead my best possible life, open wider, go even deeper inside, love more completely, and appreciate and savor the gift of every moment.

My prayer has been answered.

April 2016

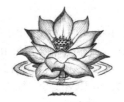

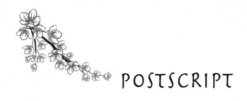

# POSTSCRIPT

The journey continues.

One week after writing the epilogue, the slow-growing follicular lymphoma diagnosis that I had danced in harmony with for almost four years without treatment mutated into a highly aggressive form. I sat with my oncologist in front of the computer screen looking at the results of the PET scan. The images looked like fireworks in a Fourth of July night sky with huge, colorful bursts of red and yellow and orange (representing bulky tumor masses) spreading throughout the liver, spleen, abdomen, femur, scapula, chest, neck areas, hilar, cervical, pelvis, and iliac and inguinal areas. Although this can be a natural transition of the slow-growing cells, she surmised that it was triggered by the huge assault on my immune system from a year of deep surgery, followed by radiation, chemotherapy, and more surgeries.

I had grand plans for the summer that certainly hadn't included a second roller coaster ride with chemotherapy and being face to face with another separate stage four diagnosis. But as the old Yiddish proverb says, "We plan, God laughs."

Life is always putting another challenge in our path, another opportunity to learn. We never know what is around the next bend or in the next moment. So, once again, I am connecting the dots of my life but trusting the bigger picture. Whatever is in front of me, I continue to bow to as my teacher.

Ironically, in the darkest hours during the stark reality of my treatment with its challenging and sometimes all-consuming side effects, I was reaching for my own words in this book as an anchor, a reminder, and a compass to all things healing. Breathe. Only right here, right now. Be still and heal. Expect a miracle. Trust. Don't know. Choose joy. Keep my heart open. It's an ever-changing sensation. This too shall pass. Everything matters. Say yes. Rest in gratitude for my life, my loving village of family and friends, and the infinite loving presence.

Always the purpose of my life is not to somehow remove all challenges but to carry my own cross with more and more grace and meaning. To rest in my essence and not in my illness. To move from my heart and not my mind. To choose love over fear.

Moment to moment, breath to breath, side effect to side effect. Once again, Team Suzette carried me on the wings of their love, compassion, generosity, positive thoughts, and prayers.

At the finish line of treatment six months later, the PET scan revealed that all is blue skies. The unwelcome cells had been sent to the far side of the moon. I picture them with a one way ticket, no return flight, and confined to a permanent residence there.

Another miracle. Amazing grace. I am blessed, humbled, joyous, and I rest in eternal gratitude.

Everything keeps changing but the part of me that never changes.

Indeed the journey is everything.

Indeed the journey never ends.

January 2017

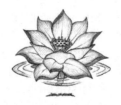

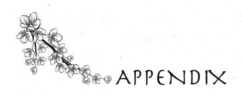 APPENDIX

## WEBSITES

TEAM SUZETTE WEBSITE: teamsuzette.weebly.com

The TEAM SUZETTE website was created by my family a few days before my initial fourteen-hour surgery as a home base to coordinate my personal care, monetary support needed during my healing journey, and to keep everyone updated on my latest progress. It developed into a place for me to share my thoughts, progress, and the endless love and gratitude I continually felt as I slowly moved through my healing journey. Many of the chapters in this book began as seeds from my updates sent out through this website. The Team Suzette website includes more specifics on the trajectory of my physical healing, pictures, and all the baby steps that became great leaps.

ART WEBSITE: suzette.cc

To view my artwork and many of the pieces created after my surgeries and treatments, please visit my art website. This website includes the first piece created six months after my surgery, entitled *The Journey is Everything*. I began to experiment with sketching, cutting, and fusing my artwork. This piece was done slowly, with adaptations from limited movement from a severed spinal accessory nerve after my sling was removed, and with a patch on one eye. Several months later, this 5' x 4.5' mixed media fine art original was created, consisting of twenty-seven panels that reflected my healing journey.

The "Rising Above" and "The Journey is Everything" link on my website shows more of the art inspired from my time in the wilderness of my healing.

# MY YONDAN ESSAY
(read three months after treatment as part of my test for my
fourth-degree black sash in tai chi at Aikido-ai of Whittier)

Six months ago, I sat in a circle on the mat and shared my upcoming surgery/treatment for highly aggressive and advanced stage four cancer with all of you. Now I will stand before you to share my understanding of yondan. This moment is not about a rush to advance in rank after an absence due to illness, nor some overwhelming and burning goal to achieve fourth degree. For me this is about the miracle of this moment in time. Sensei said he would be honored for me to do a demonstration to share my understanding of yondan level. He did not ask me six months ago nor six months from now. He was not interested in what was, what will, or what might be, but just what is so for me right now.

After my surgery, I let go of everything: how I looked, movement of my body, driving, using my eye and arms, and turning my head. Not out of a surrendering and waving of a white flag, not out of a not wanting and not out of a not caring. I let my life become a blank canvas, which stayed open to whatever new might take its place, so that whatever might return to me would be a great gift. Standing before you all right now is one of those great gifts. One may say: "She has been out of the dojo for months. How could she possibly test for fourth degree?" However, the truth is that I have been in a marathon training for yondan. My recovery has been about deep connection with the breath, moment-to-moment living, continual patience, endless meditative practice, moving slowly, staying open to allow universal healing energy to flow through me, and experiencing the power of immense love. Physically, this test may have been different six months ago. However, yondan level isn't about how athletic I can be in the form, nor how great my stamina, strength, and balance are. At this moment, I may not have a strong body, but I do have a stronger understanding of the healing force of tai chi, which moves from my quiet, still center inside, and then outward to heal me physically, emotionally, and spiritually. Blue skies far away, body deep inside.

Tai chi training can save our lives. It saved mine. Throughout my recovery, tai chi principles kept me open, relaxed, and connected to my center, yet expanding outward to everyone. They helped me, time and time again, to find the space amid the contraction, pain, and fear.

Tai chi has shown me the deep power of the breath, winding its way through all. So the inhale and exhale is all that exists: No yesterday, no tomorrow, it's just the moment and the connection to life itself. It taught me deep relaxation so I could have my face and chest bolted down in a mask, go through a radiation tunnel on a conveyor belt every day for months, be awake in the dark of the night alone, be in pain, and transform anxiety into a sense of peace. Perhaps most importantly, tai chi always reminded me that everything changes.

Yondan level is the breath. It is right here, right now. It is the stillness within the movement. Yondan is not knowing. It is loving energy. Yondan is the space that separates us and truly joins us. Yondan is the emptiness within the form. Yondan is choosing to be open time and time again. Yondan is the moment between the inhale and the exhale. Yondan is doing what I love. Yondan is both my center and universal energy. It is being more and more of who I truly am. Yondan is all that I can feel without touching. It is our spirit, which shines through our movements. Yondan is the connection to everyone and everything.

Yondan is seeking an unbroken circle between my life, my practice, and my teaching. It is about the practice of tai chi on the greater mat of the world. This flow is the advanced work of tai chi: flow from mat to life, flow in the form, and the flow that is without form. Each of our lives are our great advanced tai chi forms, which are hopefully woven together with the tai chi principles. Our lives, just like the forms, will be constantly changing if we are truly present in it. What good is our practice if it doesn't become our lives? It is said if you do what you love, you become what you love. What greater gift than to someday become tai chi?

Advancing to fourth degree is not about learning more forms, though the forms are endless and we vow to learn them all. It is the understanding that form is emptiness and emptiness is form. It is the form of my paralyzed face, but knowing that is not who I really am. It is knowing that what we are always really studying in tai chi is stillness, center, breath, balance, connection, harmony, and love.

The first movement I learned in tai chi was the movement that I had sought to execute for yondan: the integration breath. As a result of the severing of my spinal accessory nerve, which controls the neck, shoulder, and upper back, the ability to raise my right arm high enough to do a simple integration breath was a distant and very uncertain possibility. However, miracles continue to happen.

Yondan is ultimately about love and the miracle of healing. It is about your support, kindness, love, and generosity throughout my healing journey. It is my testimony that the love from and for my family, friends, and dojo have been my healing force. It reflects that aikido-ai is truly the embodiment of its name: love as the path to harmonious and healing energy. For me, yondan is ultimately about the healing, universal energy of love that connects us all.

I love you.
Suzette Hodnett
November 2014

The letter to friends and family after Tattoo's passing.

Dear friends and family,

Tattoo's lovable and strong heart took its last beat late afternoon on Wednesday. The little miracle comeback kitty has gone home. Most of you know how close to my heart I held Tattoo. This kitty, who tragically lost her mom several years ago to this same congenital heart disease, truly pulled my maternal strings to a very deep place. I feel blessed and honored to have shared part of my life with such an affectionate, loving spirit, and to have experienced her unconditional love, companionship, courage, calm in the face of health challenges, and many life lessons. Some say I took care of her throughout all her illnesses, but it was truly she who took care of me.

I will miss her warmth and purring each night, her curling up in my arms with her head on my shoulder, seeing her excited face each time I arrive home again, and the deeply peaceful time with her heavy on my chest and under my shirt that always reminded me to stop, breathe, and relax. I will miss her sitting on my lap as I talk to clients and her constant love, friendship, and healing spirit. This little gift from God named Tattoo has left an indelible mark on my heart. Love truly knows no boundaries between species.

Love,
Suzette

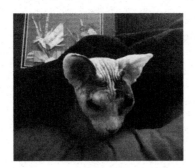

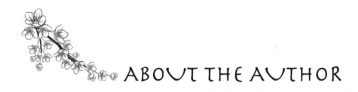

# ABOUT THE AUTHOR

Suzette Hodnett, M.S., has a background as a licensed marriage and family therapist, life coach, professional artist, and yondan tai chi instructor.

She lives in Whittier, California with a backyard menagerie of squirrels, birds, and the ever-present and ever-changing beauty of nature.

She is also the co-author of *Home Massage: Transforming Family Life Through the Healing Power of Touch*, with Chuck Fata, published by Findhorn Press, 2009.

To contact the author, please email her at
suz4thejourney@aol.com
or visit
www.thejourneyiseverything.cc

Suzette is available for speaking engagements.

COMING MAY 2021

THE SEQUEL:

# THE JOURNEY REMAINS EVERYTHING
## STILL SAYING YES